D1715157

HEALTH CARE WORK REDESIGN

SERIES ON NURSING ADMINISTRATION

SONA

SERIES ON NURSING ADMINISTRATION

An annual publication planned and administered by the University of Iowa, **SONA** addresses current and emerging issues in nursing administration. In each volume, distinguished nurse administrators and educators address the state of knowledge, future directions, and controversial questions on aspects of a particular issue and propose options for resolution. The series provides a quality resource for practicing administrators, faculty teaching nursing administration, and students in administration programs.

Volume 1: *Series on Nursing Administration*
M. Johnson, editor and J. McCloskey, chair of the board – Out of print

Volume 2: *Changing Organizational Structures.*
M. Johnson, editor and J. McCloskey, chair of the board – Out of print

Previous Volumes in the Series Available From Mosby:

Volume 3: *Delivery of Quality Health Care*
M. Johnson, editor and J. McCloskey, chair of the board

Volume 4: *Economic Myths and Realities: Doing More With No More*
M. Johnson, editor and M. Maas, chair of the board

Volume 5: *Managing Nursing Care*
K. Kelly, editor and M. Maas, chair of the board

Volume 6: *Health Care Rationing: Dilemma and Paradox*
K. Kelly, editor and M. Maas, chair of the board

Volumes Available From Sage Publications:

Volume 7: *Health Care Work Redesign*
K. Kelly, editor and M. Maas, chair of the board

Future Volumes From Sage Publications:

Volume 8: *Outcomes of Effective Management Practices*
K. Kelly, editor and M. Maas, chair of the board

Volume 9: *Nursing Roles: Evolving or Recycled*
D. Huber, editor and S. Moorhead, chair of the board

HEALTH CARE WORK REDESIGN

Kathleen Kelly
Editor

Meridean Maas
Chair of the Board

SONA 7

Series on Nursing Administration

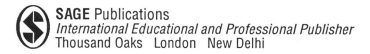

SAGE Publications
International Educational and Professional Publisher
Thousand Oaks   London   New Delhi

For information address:

SAGE Publications, Inc.
2455 Teller Road
Thousand Oaks, California 91320

SAGE Publications Ltd.
6 Bonhill Street
London EC2A 4PU
United Kingdom

SAGE Publications India Pvt. Ltd.
M-32 Market
Greater Kailash I
New Delhi 110 048 India

Printed in the United States of America

Library of Congress Cataloging-in-Publication Data

Main entry under title:

Health care work redesign / editor, Kathleen Kelly ; chair of the
    board, Meridean Maas.
         p. cm. — (Series on nursing administration; v. 7)
      Includes bibliographical references and index.
      ISBN 0-8039-7164-8 (cl. alk. paper)
      1. Nursing services—Administration.   I. Kelly, Kathleen.
    II. Maas, Meridean.   III. Series.
      [DNLM: 1. Nursing Staff, Hospital—organization & administration.
    2. Organizational Innovation.   3. Nursing Care—organization &
    administration.   4. Models, Nursing.   5. Delivery of Health Care—
    organization & administration.   W1 SE72Q v. 7 1995 / WY 105 H4337
    1995]
    RT89.H43   1995
    362.1′73′068—dc20
    DNLM/DLC
    94-44913

This book is printed on acid-free paper.

95 96 97 98 99 10 9 8 7 6 5 4 3 2 1

Production Editor: Diane S. Foster   Typesetter: Christina Hill

Contents

Series Editors' Introduction

Today's nurse executive needs to stay current in many rapidly changing areas of health care. To meet this demand, the *Series on Nursing Administration* is designed to give nursing administrators new information on current and emerging issues. Developed and managed at the University of Iowa College of Nursing, it is a quality resource for nurse executives, faculty who teach nursing administration, and students in nursing administration programs. Each year a new volume addresses the most recent issues in this discipline. Thus a subscription to the series will keep readers on the forefront of knowledge and practice.

Every nurse executive interacts with corporate management, colleagues in other settings, professional groups, the community, clients, nurse colleagues, members of other disciplines, and ancillary personnel. To stay current with developments in each of these areas the nurse executive reads journals and newsletters, attends continuing education programs, and participates in short-term executive management courses. The most effective method, however, is the sharing of concerns, experiences, and insights with peers. The *Series on Nursing Administration* formalizes the process of sharing among experts with similar concerns. In every chapter of each volume of the series, expert authors share their experiences and ideas on particular emerging issues. Busy nurse executives can conveniently and cost-effectively keep their knowledge current on a variety of topics by reading this series.

Nursing administration faculty can use the series to keep their teaching and practice alive, current, and timely. Most nursing administration programs have one or more courses that address issues in nursing management. Because these issues undergo rapid change, faculty need a flexible approach to teaching this content. This series offers the instructor maximum flexibility in selecting issues for discussion to fit the needs of a particular class. An instructor teaching a nursing management issues course can use the series as a course text. Students introduced to this series will find it a resource with ongoing value. Faculty teaching undergraduate level administration courses also may use the series to supplement an introductory text on management and leadership.

The series is unique in that it is the first annual series devoted to issues in nursing administration. To ensure that it covers current issues and provides up-to-date information, the series employs a unique publication process involving four groups: a series editor, an editorial board, the authors, and the publisher.

Editor of Volumes 1 through 4 of the series is Marion Johnson, RN, PhD, an associate professor at the University of Iowa. She has a rich practice base in nursing administration and currently teaches nursing administration at the master's level. Her background, interests, and writing skills make her eminently qualified for the job of series editor.

Kathleen C. Kelly, PhD, RN, is editor for Volumes 5 through 7 of the series. She has years of experience as a community health nursing administrator and teaches nursing administration at the master's level. She also administers the Continuing Education Program at the College of Nursing. Her background and current work provide a broad perspective on issues that are of critical importance to nurse executives and managers.

The editorial board consists of faculty teaching in the nursing administration program at Iowa and selected nurse administrators associated with the program. The board meets three to four times a year with the series editor, helps identify the emerging issues and prospective authors, and assists the editor with manuscript review. Iowa's growing program in nursing administration, including study at the doctoral level, makes this an ideal setting to support this publication.

The authors are distinguished nurse administrators, educators, and researchers chosen for their expertise in particular areas. Although authors have the freedom to pursue an issue as they choose, each is encouraged to address the state of knowledge, future directions, and the controversial questions surrounding the issue, and to propose one or more options for resolution. Beginning with Volume 7, authors are chosen by a review process following a Call for Abstracts. The Call for Abstracts is mailed and advertised in various journals and newsletters during the months of February through September each year.

The publisher of the series for Volumes 3 through 6 is Mosby-Year Book, Inc. Volumes 1 and 2 were published by Addison-Wesley. Beginning with volume 7, Sage Publications, Inc. is now publisher.

All of us involved in this series believe that it will benefit not only those who teach and practice nursing administration but the entire nursing profession and, most important, the patients we serve. We welcome your comments and suggestions.

—Joanne Comi McCloskey, PhD, RN, FAAN
Chairperson, Editorial Board, Volumes 1-4

—Meridean Maas, PhD, RN, FAAN
Chairperson, Editorial Board, Volumes 5-8

Preface

In this seventh volume of **Series on Nursing Administration,** the editors, board of directors, and contributing authors explore work redesign, a critical element in the health care industry's effort to respond to criticisms and demands from health regulatory bodies, payers, and consumers. Many chapters report on efforts to redesign health care delivery. All chapters focus on the significance of redesign to nurse managers.

Initial chapters analyze redesign and related concepts, providing convincing evidence that success in reforming health care delivery will incorporate work redesign, restructuring, and reengineering. In Chapter 1, Kohles and Donaho provide an overview of work redesign based on their unique perspective, gained in directing "Strengthening Hospital Nursing: A Program to Improve Patient Care," a project sponsored jointly by the Robert Wood Johnson Foundation and the Pew Charitable Trusts.

Redman and Ketefian expand on this overview in Chapter 2. They present issues involved in redesign, and then describe their field study and development of an instrument to measure work redesign. Tumulty offers another means of investigating work redesign, time series, in Chapter 3. The report of her findings provides an incentive for nurse managers and health organizations to consider work redesign in developing formulas for change. And in Chapter 4, Brooks and Juras describe the relationships of efficiency ratings to structural and technological characteristics, using data envelopment analysis.

Chapter 5, contributed by Coulter et al., shifts the focus to direct care and nurses' direct involvement in health care decisions. The project these authors describe demonstrates how work redesign based on case management has yielded positive results.

The perspective of those performing the activity is important to reconfiguration of any activity. In this case that is the staff nurse. In Chapter 6, Fisher et al. describe staff nurse involvement in work redesign as part of concerted efforts to empower the staff through shared governance.

Next, in Chapter 7, Peterson focuses the reader's attention on the planning and documentation elements of care delivery. Using a three-dimensional model, the author provides a foundation for addressing issues that are often time-consuming problems for nurse managers.

In Chapter 8, work redesign in process at the Tucson Medical Center, which builds on a collaborative case management framework, is presented. Del Togno-Armanasco et al. report on outcomes of a practice model that clearly differentiates tasks and responsibilities of the care team members.

Jones et al. elaborate on the patient-focused care model of service delivery in Chapter 9, describing the advantages and problems from the nurse manager perspective. Other chapters that focus on organizations and structural elements essential to work redesign follow. First, Siler et al. (Chapter 10) introduce the community design model. This model is described in the context of an academic medical center, and the term *community* is operationalized in terms of the organization's restructuring and redesigning the work of health care delivery. The next chapter shifts the scene to a small hospital serving a rural population. Zuraikat et al. (Chapter 11) describe structural changes and the reward systems in the nursing organization and provide evidence of positive outcomes of the change implemented. In Chapter 12, Stetler and Sheets share a model for differentiated staffing that distinguishes levels of practice and related competencies and activities. In the following chapter, Miller and Falco counter with the Colorado differentiated practice model, reporting on implementation in six hospitals representing both rural and urban delivery settings. Gordon et al. (Chapter 14) present a model in operation at the Johns Hopkins Hospital, based on organization, human relations, and nursing concepts. The chapter explicates the model and shares evaluation data on the dependent variables of nurses' work satisfaction, patient outcomes, and cost.

Chapters 15 and 16 emphasize evaluation of work redesign efforts. Brown analyzes the redesign successes reported in the literature as well as the factors operating within "failed" redesign efforts. Ludemann et al. describe the ongoing impact of shared governance on staff empowerment, as gauged by 6 years of program monitoring.

The final chapter by Kerfoot synthesizes the work of the book's contributing authors, benchmarking the state of work redesign in health care in hospitals during the last decade of this century. In summary, as with previous volumes, all authors strive to be proactive and futuristic rather than to dwell on past problems and success stories. The contributions in this volume have great value for practicing administrators and for students of administration science. By clarifying health care delivery problems faced today and describing science-based approaches to their solutions, these authors provide insights into tested management interventions and serve as role models for science-based practice.

CHAPTER 1

Health Care Work Redesign: An Introduction

Mary K. Kohles
Barbara A. Donaho

A profound change is happening in the delivery of health care services. Although health care leaders may not know what that change is, they do know that old visions and strategies do not seem to work anymore. They know that dreams, imagination, and innovation are encouraged to make the change happen. They know that no single theory, process, or structure will reform the environment. They know that new management competencies, collaborative interactions, and partnerships with nontraditional providers of service are needed to create integrated health care delivery systems—systems that promote services across care settings (acute, long-term, and home, emphasizing wellness and prevention as well as sickness). They know that they must embrace the principles of restructuring, reengineering, redesigning, and reinventing or be eclipsed by those leaders who understand their role as change agents for the health care environment. Nurse administrators, recognizing that innovation is a critical component of their role, are emerging as change agents; they, along with other health care leaders from many disciplines, are becoming the new trustees of the health care society. This volume provides proactive

AUTHORS' NOTE: Strengthening Hospital Nursing: A Program to Improve Patient Care is an initiative jointly sponsored by the Robert Wood Johnson Foundation and the Pew Charitable Trusts. SHNP includes 68 large and small teaching and nonteaching hospitals in 19 different states and the District of Columbia.

strategies, conceptual frameworks, and models for nurse administrators to consider as they prepare for that trustee role.

The authors of this volume address some of the perilous challenges facing nurse administrators—challenges that require imagination and creative thinking by the nurse leader as a change agent and trustee. They describe work redesign, role reconceptualization, job enrichment, competency-based performance, and transitional management strategies that must be a part of the repertoire of an effective change agent. The strategies of work, role, and delivery system redesign presented by the authors build on the conceptual and methodologic issues described by Redman and Ketefian in the second chapter. That chapter describes conceptual ingredients for work redesign, offers a macro and micro perspective, and concludes with a case study of redesign. The other chapters describe individual and organizational efforts, offering pragmatic, useful interventions to conquer challenges experienced by nurse administrators and nurse managers as they prepare the future health care workforce and implement integrated care delivery systems—systems that link care settings to form a community-based system of care.

The strategies developed throughout the chapters are proactive and interactive rather than reactive. They support meaningful changes at different levels of the organization—institutional, unit, and individual. At the institutional level, the approach is toward a comprehensive, systemic change in the organization. The focus is developing a fundamental philosophy for patient-centered care throughout the organization. Interventions stem from the question, Why does the organization do what it does—why does it exist?

At the unit level, the interventions are work redesign, role reconceptualization, job enrichment, differentiated practice, shared governance, and self-managed units. The resulting models or archetypes are designed to accommodate the needs of specific patient groups, use manpower and other resources efficiently, promote operational flexibility, improve quality, and control or reduce cost. At the individual level, "empowerment for redesign" is described from a staff nurse perspective. Whether the innovation occurs at the organizational, unit, or individual level, a set of standards or basic premises is identified, thereby setting the framework for evaluation strategies.

Evaluation is an essential component of redesigning/restructuring efforts. The evaluation design may not take on the characteristics of the traditional experimental design, but rather that of action learning/action research. The evaluation design has to adapt to a constantly changing environment, produce useful knowledge derived from real-world practice, and allow for a better understanding of what is happening during restructuring. The principles of action learning/action research allow for flexibility and timely use of information. Case studies, interviews, surveys, meeting minutes, anecdotal stories, and operational management reports are the data sources for action learning. The structure and data collection processes for action learning can be very simple or extremely sophisticated, depending on the intended use of the study results. The authors show, by their redesigning/restructuring efforts, that nurse administrators must look to the field of organizational development to learn and use principles of work and role redesign, systems thinking, transitional management, interactive processes, and action learning.

STRENGTHENING HOSPITAL NURSING PROGRAMS: CONCEPTS IN ACTION

Nurse leaders participating in the national Strengthening Hospital Nursing Program (SHNP) can affirm the importance of using principles and theories of organizational development before undertaking restructuring projects such as work flow processes, productivity management initiatives, system/operational reengineering, role reconceptualization, and organizational culture change efforts. Like the authors of this volume, SHNP participants are designing work environments to optimally use nurses and other human resources; implementing integrated, patient-centered care delivery systems through the coordinated efforts of all care providers, including nurses, physicians, support staff, and other professionals; creating opportunities for career enrichment and advancement for the professional nurse; and using action learning as their primary evaluation design. Patient-centered care is one of the constants between the efforts of the contributing authors and the redesign efforts of SHNP. Patient-centered care in the context of SHNP means that the delivery of services is designed to meet the needs of the patient rather than the needs of a department or discipline. Patient services take place in the environment most germane to the patient, and services are provided by the most appropriate care provider. Patient-centered care values the patient and patient's family as significant to care/case management processes.

Although each author's report on redesign is unique to his or her environment, the reader will note similarities in their visions, processes, structures, and desired outcomes for redesign. The models involve multiple disciplines, striving for interdependent relationships; commitment from key stakeholders such as executive leadership, trustees, physicians, nurses, and other disciplines; and a shared vision for improving patient care services and enhancing the quality work life of care providers. Implementation usually begins with a specific unit or department, serving as the pilot or demonstration. A structured demonstration, with defined goals, objectives, and desired outcomes, sets the stage for assessing what is working well and what is not working well. The authors advise that the nurse administrator should anticipate resistance and dissatisfaction during the early phases of demonstration. For example, differentiating skills and tasks and dividing them differently between professionals and technical workers can result in questions about job security. The "what is in it for me" question usually surfaces at some point in the process. Whatever the cause, resistance must be acknowledged and dealt with early on, or the change may be sabotaged before it has an opportunity to create improvement for patients, nurses, other care providers, and the organization.

Before you, the reader, begin exploring the chapters in this volume, you are invited to imagine the types of nurses and other workers that you think match the needs of the future health care system—the health care system desired for the 21st century. Imagine the competencies needed by nurses, other professionals, and the support staff. Ask yourself what relationships need to form and develop in order to ensure those competencies. Consider the merit of involving schools of nursing and allied health programs in your design processes; forming partnerships with university and community colleges; establishing relationships with elementary schools and high schools; and consulting with the contributors of this volume. Identify your responsibility as a nurse leader in the process for creating roles that reach across a continuum of service or care settings. Imagine how your contribution in redesign can meet patient needs for future generations, and what the new designs, roles, and delivery methods may mean to your pursuit to be a trustee for the health care systems of the future.

CHAPTER 2

Defining and Measuring
Work Redesign: A Field Study

Richard Redman
Shaké Ketefian

This chapter examines conceptual and definitional issues in work redesign, with particular emphasis on work redesign efforts in nursing. A field study and a newly developed instrument to measure nursing work redesign efforts are described. Baseline data provide insights to various approaches taken to work redesign and the considerable variation that exists. Implications for work redesign efforts are presented to guide nurse administrators in the future.

AUTHORS' NOTE: The authors express appreciation to the members of the research team of a large project of which this study is a part. Specifically, we are pleased to acknowledge the contribution of the following individuals at the University of Michigan Medical Center: Sheri R. Dufek, RN, MSA, Associate Hospital Administrator/Director of Nursing, Operating Rooms; Debra A. Finch, RN, BSN, Assistant Director of Clinical Programs and Research; Beverly Jones, RN, MPH, Chief of Nursing Affairs; Joan O. Robinson, RN, MS, Associate Hospital Administrator/Director of Nursing, Ambulatory Care; and Carol D. Spengler, RN, PhD, Associate Hospital Administrator/Director of Nursing, Pediatric, Perinatal, and Psychiatric Nursing. In addition, we are grateful for the assistance of Erna-Lynne Bogue, RN, doctoral candidate in sociology at the University of Michigan; Cheryl D. Rorie, RN, doctoral candidate at the University of Michigan School of Nursing; and Patricia Williams, RN, MS, Computer Systems Consultant, Pediatric, Perinatal, and Psychiatric Nursing. Requests for the Work Redesign Questionnaire may be addressed to Dr. Redman at the University of Michigan, School of Nursing, 400 North Ingalls, Ann Arbor, MI 48109-0482.

The rapid changes in health care and the reimbursement system in the past decade, along with the frequent recurrence of nursing shortages, have challenged health care administrators to develop innovative strategies to meet patient care needs while containing costs. Work redesign, in its various forms, has evolved as one such strategy.

In an undertaking of work redesign, the many meanings of the term *work* take on increased importance. Hall (1986) defined *work* as an activity that produces something of value, the means to earning a living. It has various synonyms: *Production, effort, labor,* and *employment* are examples. However work is defined, it is viewed as a purposeful activity. It may not matter whether the work has more meaning to the individual who performs it or to others who benefit from it until an attempt is made to redesign it.

Just as the meanings of work are varied, the approaches to changing how it is performed also are varied. Examples of the approaches include work/job redesign, work/job restructuring, redesigning hospital nursing practice, redesigning patient care, job enrichment and redesign, nursing role redesign, and restructuring nursing care delivery systems. What do these terms mean? How do we recognize them when we see them? How are they measured? These issues can influence how work redesign efforts are implemented and evaluated.

Work redesign efforts are prevalent in nursing and health care institutions. Yet there is considerable lack of conceptual and methodological clarity regarding what these entail, what the expected outcomes are, and how goal achievement is evaluated.

The purpose of this chapter is to examine the various conceptual meanings of the terms related to work redesign. One method of operationalizing a work redesign effort will be described, and the methods used to measure the goals and strategies for this work redesign will be discussed. Special emphasis will be placed on the challenges related to measuring work redesign. Finally, implications for future work redesign efforts in nursing will be presented.

PERSPECTIVES ON WORK REDESIGN

Approaches may begin at the top levels of the organization and disseminate down to the production levels or may begin at the bottom and work up. Whether a macro or micro focus is utilized, it is recognized that redesigns have far-reaching effects beyond the particular departments or roles that may have been redesigned. The redesign efforts can achieve both intended and unintended results.

The goals of work redesign are typically the same, whether approached from a macro or micro perspective. Generally, organizations undertake these efforts to reduce costs, increase operational flexibility, improve quality, strengthen organizational integration, and improve efficiency. Any particular goal may be the primary objective, or a combination of goals may be of interest. These goals can pertain in any type of industry, including service industries such as health care.

Work redesign efforts draw upon theories, models, and tools from several disciplines: management sciences, engineering, sociology, psychology, and economics. No one theory is identified as the best framework. However, general systems theory appears frequently as one theoretical referent. The scope or level of redesign is important to consider: macro, or whole system, versus micro, or individual work unit level.

The related literature can be conceptualized on a macro level in terms of broad system redesign or narrowly on a micro level in terms of redesigning the specific work of nurses (work and job redesign). Each will be described in terms of nature and goals. The distinctions between these classifications are not always as clear as the terms would imply, and in practice there are overlapping elements.

System Redesign

Macro-level approaches encompass restructuring major divisions within an organization with the intent of changing several or all subsystems. At the organizational level, the focus is generally on increasing the productivity of the organization as a system, improving the quality of the goods and services produced, and improving overall system coordination.

Various authors present their perspectives on redesigning the nursing care delivery system or the manner in which patient care is delivered as part of an overall effort to redesign the organization. Dienemann and Gessner (1992) described an approach that involves redesigning the larger context within which care is delivered. According to a systems theory view that considers organizations as interactive, interdependent entities, all elements of a system are affected by a redesign effort. Both management and professional groups are involved; "The emphasis is on management of work flow and standards of practice as a context for professional practice" (p. 255). The goal is to create an environment in which professionals make autonomous decisions within expected parameters of quality, cost management, and productivity (Sheridan, Vredenburgh, & Abelson, 1984).

A number of models of system redesign are identified from the literature. Generally these use some form of case management, with variations. Specific models are reported by Zander (1988) for the New England Medical Center Hospital, Loveridge, Cummings, and O'Malley (1988) for Sharp Medical

Center, Del Togno-Armanasco, Olivas, and Harter (1989) and others for Tucson Medical Center, and Brett and Tonges (1990) for Robert Wood Johnson University Hospital. These settings use various modalities of care and nursing assignments. Fralic (1992) described the creation of new practice models as well as new roles within the Robert Wood Johnson University Hospital. Here, too, the impetus seems to have been pressures with regard to nurse availability and affordability, and the need to make systems more effective for patient care delivery.

Dienemann and Gessner (1992) also included total quality management (TQM) as another instance of total restructuring of the system and the way in which care is delivered. This approach, based on systems theory, involves a paradigm shift, is customer driven, and uses a continuous quality improvement process.

Although the typical system redesign approach emphasizes restructuring macro-level components of the organization, newer approaches are sensitive to the individuals in the organization as well. Morris and Brandon (1993) discussed a "reengineering" approach that begins with a fundamental understanding of how processes work in the organization and how the work groups perform. They felt it is erroneous to define jobs and positions solely on the basis of the work that needs to be done and to exclude consideration of the individuals who perform those jobs. Thus restructuring efforts will only be effective when organizational, group, and individual behavior is considered. Reengineering results in an interactive approach blending both macro and micro strategies.

Smeltzer (1992) recommended that hospitals engage in work restructuring to address cost, availability of professional workers, and enhancement of patient and nurse satisfaction. She took a multidisciplinary view of the effort and the need to analyze specific job categories, so that as work is restructured, all employees are utilized to their fullest.

Strasen (1989) described her conceptions of redesigning patient care as a means of cost saving to integrate functions of respiratory therapy into nursing and to integrate housekeepers into the patient care team. These redesigns are meant to eliminate duplication, increase efficiency, and make the nurse the coordinator for all patient care activities. Thus although the term *redesign* appears to classify this author's work within system redesign, the intent is more aligned with work redesign.

Work and Job Redesign

Hackman and Oldham (1980) provided a conceptual framework for work redesign that supports this work redesign effort. Their job characteristics model (JCM) is based on behavioral and sociotechnical concepts. Their research tested the hypothesis that enhancing the psychological states of workers leads to high work effectiveness. The JCM components are discussed in more detail in the description of this field study.

The micro-level focus of work redesign begins with an examination of job or position characteristics and requirements and the needs of employees who fill those jobs. Jobs can be understood and categorized in a number of different ways: tasks performed; worker skill, knowledge, and qualifications; rewards obtained; motivational needs of the individual; degree of autonomy or discretion in the job. Nystrom (1981) described universal characteristics of jobs: variety, autonomy, required interactions, required skill and knowledge, and responsibility. These dimensions vary from job to job. When redesigning work from this perspective, it is essential that employee needs and perceptions be considered along with the requirements of the organization. In fact, redesign is often referred to as *enrichment* because jobs are redesigned in such a way as to enhance the fit between work and the employee. A choice of approaches to work redesign exists and ranges from job rotation and enlargement to complete redefinition of traditional roles and work requirements (Campbell & Campbell, 1990).

Madden and Lawrenz (1990) viewed work redesign in health care from a multidisciplinary framework and approached restructuring the nursing work environment by using a sociotechnical systems model. In this approach, people and technology are linked in ways such that both are optimized. The redesign efforts include multiple focused interventions that range from redesigned jobs and reward systems to creation of work groups that share decision making about how work is best accomplished.

According to Dienemann and Gessner (1992), job design, which they distinguished from systems redesign, is a bottom-up approach focusing on shaping jobs to optimize productivity. Job enrichment is designed to achieve the following: generate organizational commitment, allow for differences in positions with different competence, support professional collaborative practice, and involve nurses in broader institutional and policy-making activities. Job design models discussed are primary and total care, clinical ladders, differentiated practice, Partners in Practice, and shared governance. Each of these models or strategies is responsive to different unit, organizational, or professional needs.

Cunningham and Eberle (1990) took a different view of job/work redesign. They began with the contention that traditional approaches to designing work can adversely affect organizations, and employee motivation and satisfaction. Thus alternative ways of designing jobs should be explored. They reviewed four theoretical perspectives, each of which makes different assumptions about individuals and the cultural context of the organization.

1. *Herzberg's (1966) two-factor theory of job enrichment.* In this theory, factors that produce job satisfaction and motivation are different from the factors that lead to job dissatisfaction. Achievement, recognition, the work, responsibility, and advancement are growth and motivation factors, whereas institutional policy, administration, technical supervision, and work conditions are hygiene factors that can cause dissatisfaction. Reducing job dissatisfaction will not by itself increase growth and motivation. Those elements that enhance job satisfaction and motivation are viewed as factors that enrich a job and should be stressed during job redesign.

2. *The job characteristics model.* Hackman and Oldham's (1980) research provided the basis for this approach to investigating the effectiveness of work redesign. This model is based on the notion that jobs have core characteristics, that people respond differently to the same job, and that work can be structured in such a way that it can be performed well and be satisfying to the employee. Five job characteristics have been identified: task identity, task significance, skill variety, autonomy, and job-based feedback.

3. *Japanese-style management.* This is based on norms of harmony and organizational cohesiveness. Employees are socialized extensively and are transferred from job to job to learn new skills. Such rotation builds experience, enables the grooming of future managers, immerses the employee in the culture and philosophy of the company, and enables a certain degree of mobility in an environment in which promotional opportunities are limited.

4. *Quality of work life.* There are several approaches in this model but no standard set of principles, for these have to be tailored to the needs of the individuals and those of the technology. These approaches replace terms such as *work design* and *sociotechnical design.* The job designs evolve as new technologies come to the fore and as individual capacities change. Any subject of concern to the employees can be addressed, including wages, hours, and other work conditions.

IMPLICATIONS OF VARIOUS PERSPECTIVES

Each theory and model illustrates a different conceptual view of work redesign. Some emphasize the work that needs to be accomplished, whereas others focus on the structure or the jobs that have been defined to carry out that work. A further distinction focuses on the impact that the redesigned work or job has on the individual who carries it out. Different conceptual definitions result.

The conceptual differences in the various models suggest different strategies for work redesign and different types of outcomes that might be accomplished. In nursing, these differences range from restructuring the organizational approaches for delivering nursing care to redesigning roles for nurses and other personnel involved in delivering patient care services. The strategies and the outcomes for a particular work redesign effort necessarily vary with the basic assumptions made about work and employees.

These differences become very apparent when attempts are made to operationalize a work redesign effort in an organization and measure its effects. The term *work redesign* often is employed to cover a variety of programmatic efforts that include specific goals and strategies. Although the goals for work redesign may be clear, the strategies for accomplishing those goals may be less clear. This can be exaggerated in a decentralized organization when approaches to work redesign are individualized and unit based. The lack of conceptual clarity, as well as variation in approaches for implementation, presents a number of challenges when one is trying to measure the effects of a work redesign effort. Further, no instrument is available to evaluate work redesign implementation. A new instrument was developed for this study. A case study of one effort provides insights about these methodologic challenges.

CASE STUDY OF WORK REDESIGN:
DEFINITION AND OPERATIONALIZATION

A major field study, currently under way, has underscored definitional and measurement issues concerning work redesign in nursing. One component of this study has been to implement a major work redesign program that focuses on the role of the registered nurse. In this section, the field study will be described briefly. The work redesign effort will be described, and the Work Redesign Questionnaire (a measurement instrument that was developed to evaluate progress toward accomplishing work redesign goals) will be presented along with reliability and validity data. Results to date on the work redesign program will be discussed and analyzed.

Field Study

The setting in which the field study is being conducted is a large, tertiary medical center. The purpose of the project is to measure the effects of two specific administrative interventions on nurses and patients. The two major administrative interventions selected were work redesign and the implementation of a shared governance structure. Three years earlier, the entire institution began a total quality management program. The field study interventions were developed within this context.

The specific goals of the study were to improve cost efficiency, nurse satisfaction, and patient and family satisfaction. Two assumptions were made: Decisions concerning patient care and service should be made by those who are closest to the work, and participation of those most affected by the redesign process results in the best solution and greatest empowerment.

Although some authors subsume shared governance under the broader umbrella of work redesign, within the institution where the study was conducted shared governance and work redesign are two distinctive initiatives. This chapter features the work redesign portion of the study.

Conceptual and Operational Definitions

After the theoretical literature on work redesign was reviewed, the job characteristics model (JCM) (Hackman & Oldham, 1980) appeared to be the most appropriate for the purpose at hand, fit best with the philosophical orientation of the investigators, and had the advantage of being accompanied by a valid and reliable measure. Hackman and Oldham referred to the JCM as a hybrid model based on the behavioral and sociotechnical approaches. Behavioral approaches hold that work effectiveness is enhanced if employees have jobs that are complex, meaningful, and challenging instead of simple and repetitive. The sociotechnical systems approach accepts the major premises of the behavioral approach but goes beyond them and addresses the importance of group relationships and organization-environment transactions in forming effective work groups.

Hackman and Oldham (1980) theorized that jobs have certain core characteristics that lead to critical psychological states, which in turn lead to certain outcomes. In this framework, the job characteristics of skill variety, task identity, and task significance lead the employee to experience the work as meaningful. The characteristic of autonomy leads to the experience of responsibility for the outcomes of the work. The characteristic of feedback from the job itself leads to knowledge of the actual results of the work activities. These psychological states are expected to lead to the following outcomes: high internal work motivation, high growth satisfaction, high general job satisfaction, and high work effectiveness. Three variables are thought to moderate the relationships between job characteristics and psychological states, and between psychological states and outcomes. These variables are knowledge and skill, growth need strength, and context satisfaction (such as pay and job security) (Hackman & Oldham, 1980, p. 90). The Job Diagnostic Survey (JDS; Hackman & Oldham, 1975) is the standardized instrument that is used to measure the various components of the Hackman and Oldham model. The JDS was one of the standardized instruments administered to all participants in the field study.

This theoretical perspective has spurred much research in the social sciences, and many of the propositions have been tested. The main criticism has been that there is scant evidence regarding the hypothesis that the enhancement of psychological states leads to high work effectiveness.

The research team integrated components of the Hackman and Oldham model with the perspective of Madden and Lawrenz (1990), which focuses on sociotechnical approaches. For purposes of this research, work redesign is viewed as involving the restructuring of work roles and/or the work environment for the purpose of improving the efficiency and effectiveness of the patient care delivery system. The primary focus is on nursing practice. Work redesign is viewed within a sociotechnical framework, valuing the impact of the work and its redesign in terms of social aspects, namely, the worker and the work group, as well as organizational and technologic aspects. A multidisciplinary, multifaceted, interactive approach is being used to redesign the work of nursing, although the specific strategies utilized vary depending on the type of patient care services provided and the needs of each work group. Although the strategies to redesign work vary, the primary interest is in the effects of the redesign effort on nurses, patients, and families.

In the field study, work redesign is measured in terms of the outcome of the work redesign efforts and the impact of that redesign on the individuals who are performing the work. Outcomes include actual or substantive changes in the roles or the work environment at the nursing unit level as well as the impact of the redesigned work on the nurses, their roles, the tasks they perform, and the working environment in which they carry out their roles and tasks. An instrument to measure the work redesign goals and progress toward their accomplishment was developed due to the lack of such instruments in the literature.

Methodology

Employing a field study design, data were gathered on all relevant variables for both work redesign and shared governance, representing baseline measures, prior to the outset of the formal interventions. These relevant variables include levels of professionalism, components of professional practice, job characteristics, affective responses, values and culture of the organization, and organizational commitment. All registered nurses in all areas of the institution with regular appointments, full or part time ($N = 2,200$), were invited to participate. Approval from the Human Subjects Review Committee as well as appropriate administrative personnel within the institution was obtained. Participation was voluntary, and completing the questionnaires was interpreted as consent on the part of individual nurses. All inpatient, operating room, and ambulatory units were included; 1,030 registered nurses completed the study instruments, for an overall response rate of 51%.

Several standardized instruments were administered to the individual nurse subjects. In addition, a number of instruments were designed specifically for the purposes of the study because standardized measures currently do not exist. These included measures for professional practice and decision making in nursing (shared governance) and nursing work redesign.

A work redesign process was developed for use within the institution, but units were encouraged to develop their own goals and specific strategies for achieving those goals. This approach supported the above assumptions and was based on the recognition that patient and staff requirements and needs varied widely across the units and that work redesign activities had to be responsive to these needs.

Instrument Development

The purpose of the instrument was to measure work redesign activities on units and to evaluate progress toward work redesign goals following a designated period allowed for implementation. During the initial phase of item development, a wide variety of work redesign goals and concepts likely to be used across the institution were compiled. These were then analyzed. Three distinctive notions emerged from the analysis of the initial input. It was clear that specified goals were being pursued, that for each goal specific strategies and approaches were being used, and that progress in implementing each strategy or approach varied greatly across the institution. Therefore, the instrument was designed to tap these three dimensions.

The questionnaire is an objective, paper-and-pencil test that is easy to complete and takes about 20 minutes. Six goals are identified: use of alternative care providers; elimination of non-nursing tasks from the registered nurse's role; responses to unexpected staffing needs; improving systems and streamlining operations; consolidating units, or work of units; and utilizing technology to enhance patient outcomes and make the work of nurses easier. Each goal is accompanied with 4 to 10 relevant strategies. For each of the listed strategies, an implementation scale follows in the form of a visual analogue.

For each goal respondents check yes or no to indicate if this is a unit goal. If they check yes, they are asked to check which of the relevant strategies they utilized (yes or no), and, for those strategies selected, to mark on a visual analogue scale to what degree the unit is implementing that particular strategy. The continuum for the visual analogue scale has the anchors *have not started* on the left and *implementation is complete* on the right. Each scale is 100 mm long.

Two small pilot studies were conducted to determine inclusiveness, clarity, and representativeness of items. A number of revisions were made. One pilot was followed by a focus group with 12 respondents. A number of significant revisions following this discussion led to a revised structure of the instrument that would make it easier to respond to.

Reliability. Reliability analyses included an assessment of whether the responses to the questions were such that informed raters would agree on the status of work redesign for the unit. The managers of seven units were asked to complete a copy of the questionnaire and, at the same time, assign another staff member involved in the work redesign process to independently complete another copy. These pairs of raters were asked not to discuss their responses with each other until after they had completed the form. Three indices of interrater reliability were computed for the seven participating units, as follows: agreement of raters on goals, 76.2%; agreement of raters on strategies being utilized, 69.2%; agreement of raters on implementation of strategies, 86.8%.

Validity. Face and content validity were established through the expertise of the registered nurses expressed during participation in the focus groups and pilot testing. The instrument went through several drafts as wording and content were revised to meet stated criteria. During its use, considerable variation in goal selection and implementation across the institution was found and judged by nurse administrators and managers to capture quite closely the differences known to exist in the actual approaches to work redesign and the degree of progress in implementation. Thus the instrument appeared to capture the major dimensions of work redesign in this institution adequately and was sensitive to known variation. Discriminant validity was judged to be adequate.

Data Management

Scoring. For each goal or strategy identified by a yes response, a score of 1 was assigned; 0 was assigned for a no response. The visual analogue for implementation (on a 100-mm scale) was scored by a ruler to determine the location of the response. For each questionnaire, three scores were derived: For goals, yes responses were added; for strategies, yes responses were added; for implementation, the millimeters checked on the visual analogue were added to arrive at total scores.

Analyses. Analyzed data were at two levels, individual and unit. Descriptive analyses on work redesign goals and strategies were conducted at the unit level to provide comparisons across the organization. Additional analyses were conducted to examine characteristics of individual nurses as measured by the JDS. In order to maintain the nurse as the unit of analysis, the aggregate unit scores on work redesign were ascribed to individual nurses from each respective unit. The analyses consisted of correlations and analysis of variance.

Results

The managers of units within the institution were asked to complete the work redesign questionnaire for the unit. Baseline data on all 55 units of the institution were obtained. Two units did not select any goals and were deleted from subsequent analyses.

Description of the Status of Work Redesign Within Units. Summary results for goals and strategies are presented in Table 2.1. The number and percentage of the 53 units that selected each goal and its relevant strategies are presented first. Next, the mean implementation scores computed from the visual analogues for all strategies chosen are presented. These range from 0 to 100, with higher scores indicating a greater degree of implementation achieved for that strategy. Finally, an overall mean for progress toward accomplishing that goal, computed as the mean of all implementation scores, is presented. The mean number of work redesign goals per unit was 4.1, indicating that multiple goals were selected by a unit to address work redesign on that unit. Similarly, the number and types of strategies chosen varied, depending on the nature of the work on a unit and the type of clients served.

Comparison of Work Redesign Across Units and Clinical Services. The total number of goals and strategies selected across all settings and clinical specialties was examined for differences using analysis of variance. Although variation in goals and strategies was noted, none of the differences were statistically significant. Progress toward implementation varied considerably, however, with statistically significant differences in five of the six goals (all but the consolidation goal). The adult medical/surgical and ambulatory units consistently demonstrated further progress toward work redesign efforts.

A primary focus was on the components of nursing jobs: skill variety, task identity and significance, feedback from the job, and autonomy. When these various components of nursing jobs were examined using analysis of variance, statistically significant differences were found consistently between ambulatory and inpatient units in terms of these job components. Correlations between the work redesign goals and strategies and job components were carried out to provide further insights about the degree of difference that existed across units and specialties. Statistically significant differences were

TABLE 2.1   Frequency and Percentage of Goals/Strategies of Work Redesign, and
Mean Implementation of Strategies, by Units ($N = 53$)

Goals/Strategies	Units Choosing Number	Units Choosing Percentage	Mean Implementation of Strategies Chosen	Overall Mean Progress
Eliminate Non-Nursing Tasks	48	90.6		48
Evaluate activities	42	79.2	56	
Reallocate job responsibilities	42	79.2	43	
Delegate	41	77.3	46	
Review workload patterns	37	68.9	51	
Change assignment patterns	35	66.0	44	
Revise scheduling of non-RNs	30	56.6	48	
Utilize Alternate Care Providers	47	88.7		
a. Provider type:				59.3
Registered nurses	27	50.9	80	
Nursing assistants	27	50.9	69	
Aides	26	49.0	59	
LPNs	23	43.4	73	
Technicians	16	30.2	33	
Medical assistants	8	15.1	42	
b. What is being achieved:				42.3
Use appropriate work for task	46	86.8	49	
Improve process and efficiency	38	71.7	45	
Increase satisfaction	36	67.9	48	
Increase support staff	32	60.4	57	
Review work process	25	47.2	52	
Eliminate redundancy	19	35.8	47	
Increase use of technology	8	15.1	33	
Reduce cost	6	11.3	48	
Improve Systems	40	75.0		37.8
Reallocate job responsibilities	35	66.0	42	
Revise mode of care delivery	32	60.4	39	
Eliminate redundancy	26	49.0	35	
Revise work methods	24	45.3	36	
Eliminate tasks	20	37.7	37	
Respond to Unexpected Staffing Needs	33	62.3		55.5
Redistribute tasks	31	58.5	45	
Implement scheduling pattern of RNs	29	54.7	56	
Add staffing to meet increased activity	21	39.6	57	
Implement on-call systems	7	13.2	64	
Utilize Technology	33	62.3		40.5
Save staff time/effort	28	52.8	38	
Improve timeliness of data	24	45.3	40	
Improve overall quality of data	24	45.3	40	

(Continued)

TABLE 2.1 (Continued)

Goals/Strategies	Units Choosing Number	Units Choosing Percentage	Mean Implementation of Strategies Chosen	Overall Mean Progress
Increase safety of patients and staff	24	45.3	40	
Improve accuracy of data	23	43.4	37	
Decrease number of steps in care activities	23	43.4	37	
Integrate data from multiple sources	23	43.4	43	
Enable access to data as needed	20	37.7	38	
Enable transport of patients	20	37.7	39	
Support individualized patient education	19	35.8	53	
Consolidate Units or Work of Units	16	30.2		50.5
Sharing resources/services across units/programs	13	24.5	5	
Streamline management and operations	11	20.7	66	
Consolidate units or programs	9	17.0	67	
Streamline professional services	6	11.3	64	

found in a number of dimensions. Again, consistent and striking differences were found between ambulatory units and selected inpatient units. Negative correlations (ranging from $-.14$ to $-.49$) were quite common in adult medical/surgical inpatient and ambulatory units, and modest positive correlations (ranging from $.12$ to $.26$) were common in pediatric, perinatal, and psychiatric inpatient units. For example, higher scores on job characteristics, such as skill variety and task significance, were negatively correlated with the number of goals and strategies selected in medical/surgical and ambulatory settings; task significance was negatively correlated and skill variety was positively correlated in pediatrics, perinatal, and psychiatric units. These consistent patterns suggest that components of the nursing jobs vary considerably across specialty and setting and that the direction of these relationships also varies.

DISCUSSION AND CONCLUSIONS

The data on work design efforts to date provide interesting insights for the application of work redesign concepts and approaches in nursing. Even though these data are defined as baseline to an evaluation effort, patterns and issues emerge. Many of these issues are consistent with those discussed in the literature.

The number of goals and strategies per unit suggest that work redesign is a multifaceted, complex effort rather than a singular activity to accomplish a particular objective. In addition, the types of goals and strategies varied considerably across units, indicating that needs and approaches will vary in a highly decentralized organization.

It is apparent that work redesign holds different meanings. Although the instrument and data collection were intended to provide baseline measures before work redesign efforts were launched, the results indicate that considerable progress toward work redesign goals was already under way. At the outset of the formal and official beginning of work redesign, no progress on implementation was expected on strategies; however, data show that this is not the case, and much effort and progress had been ongoing prior to data collection. It appears difficult to view work redesign as a distinct entity or program with clearly identified beginning and ending points. This is no doubt especially true in the rapidly changing health care environment, in which nurse managers initiate a number of improvements to improve efficiency and effectiveness of patient care systems even though a formal work redesign program may not have been initiated.

Work redesign is also viewed differently and defined in various ways by different individuals. Even though certain efforts may not have been formally viewed as "work redesign," the efforts already were under way as evidenced by the progress toward completion of various goals. The reliability measures of the instrument also suggest definitional problems, even when knowledgeable individuals are members of the same organizational unit working on common goals. The term *work redesign* suggests a formal effort; in reality, it may be an ongoing amorphous activity that is a part of the larger change efforts under way in most organizations.

It is clear that differences exist in both job characteristics and work redesign efforts when clinical specialty and setting are taken into consideration. Variations across units and settings were apparent. Work redesign efforts were conceived as highly individualized efforts, with each unit having authority to determine its own goals and methods. This was necessary because the needs of clients and therefore the nature of work, varied so greatly. The data suggest that work redesign should not be approached uniformly relative to specialty of nursing practice. Consistent differences in job characteristics between ambulatory and inpatient practice suggest that work components and needs are quite different between these settings. Furthermore, some differences in the inpatient areas were noted, suggesting that differences do exist in work redesign needs in adult medical/surgical units versus pediatric, perinatal, and psychiatric specialty areas. Attention to the unique needs of various specialties and units would appear to be a very important consideration for any work redesign effort.

Clarity in conceptual and operational definitions in a work redesign program takes on additional value in nursing practice. The broader work redesign literature indicates that individuals interact with their work roles and responsibilities in ways that can have a major impact on the motivation of individuals as well as their productivity. Given the variation in the field study data, two additional critical factors in nursing work redesign would appear to be clinical specialty and setting. The final study data, after work redesign efforts are viewed as completed, should provide additional and important insights in terms of how these factors actually influence work redesign efforts and their success.

REFERENCES

Brett, J. L. L., & Tonges, M. C. (1990). Restructuring patient care delivery: Evaluation of the ProAct(TM) model. *Nursing Economics $, 8*(1), 36-44.

Campbell, J. P., & Campbell, R. J. (1990). *Productivity in organizations: New perspectives from industrial and organizational psychology.* San Francisco: Jossey-Bass.

Cunningham, J. B., & Eberle, T. (1990, February). A guide to job enrichment and redesign. *Personnel, 67,* 56-61.

Del Togno-Armanasco, V., Olivas, G., & Harter, S. (1989). Developing an integrated nursing case management model. *Nursing Management, 20*(10), 26-29.

Dienemann, J., & Gessner, T. (1992). Restructuring nursing care delivery systems. *Nursing Economics $, 10*(4), 253-258, 310.

Fralic, M. F. (1992). Creating new practice models and designing new roles: Reflections and recommendations. *Journal of Nursing Administration, 22*(6), 7-8.

Hackman, J. R., & Oldham, G. R. (1975). Development of the Job Diagnostic Survey. *Journal of Applied Psychology, 60*(2), 159-170.

Hackman, J. R., & Oldham, G. R. (1980). *Work redesign.* Reading, MA: Addison-Wesley.

Hall, R. H. (1986). *Dimensions of work.* Beverly Hills, CA: Sage.

Herzberg, S. (1966). *Work and the nature of man.* Cleveland, OH: World.

Loveridge, C. E., Cummings, S. H., & O'Malley, J. (1988). Developing case management in a primary nursing system. *Journal of Nursing Administration, 18*(10), 36-39.

Madden, M. J., & Lawrenz, E. (1990). Work redesign. In G. G. Meyer, M. J. Madden, & E. Lawrenz (Eds.), *Patient care delivery models* (pp. 3-12). Rockville, MD: Aspen.

Morris, D., & Brandon, J. (1993). *Re-engineering your business.* New York: McGraw-Hill.

Nystrom, P. C. (1981). Designing jobs and assigning employees. In P. C. Nystrom & W. H. Starbuck (Eds.), *Handbook of organizational design* (Vol. 2, pp. 272-301). New York: Oxford University Press.

Sheridan, J. E., Vredenburgh, D. J., & Abelson, M. A. (1984). Contextual model of leadership influence in hospital units. *Academy of Management Journal, 27*(1), 57-78.

Smeltzer, C. H. (1992). Work restructuring: After the decision is made. *Journal of Nursing Administration, 22*(11), 5-6.

Strasen, L. (1989). Redesigning patient care to empower nurses and increase productivity. *Nursing Economics, 7*(1), 32-35.

Zander, K. (1988). Nursing case management: Strategic management of cost and quality outcomes. *Journal of Nursing Administration, 18*(5), 23-30.

CHAPTER 3

Nurse Manager Role Redesign

Gail Tumulty

The nurse manager role is pivotal to control of cost and quality in the acute care setting. The theory and process of nurse manager role redesign are discussed in conjunction with a redesign project that is being studied using a time series design. The results indicate that positive changes in the quality of work life for the nurse manager, with subsequent positive outcomes for the hospital, can be achieved through carefully redesigned roles.

The restructuring of reimbursement systems coupled with a resurgence of shortages in health care personnel has created a demand for the development and implementation of innovative nursing roles and care delivery systems. Alternative modes of care delivery and redesigned roles are needed to enhance retention and delivery of high-quality care (Moritz, Hinshaw, & Heinrich, 1989).

The nurse manager role in the acute care setting has long been considered one of pivotal importance for the hospital. The American Academy of Nursing's landmark publication, Magnet Hospitals: Attraction and Retention of Professional Nurses (McClure, Poulin, Sovie, & Wandelt, 1983) cited nurse managers (head nurses) as a major factor influencing the attraction and retention of nurses. In a follow-up to the Magnet Hospital Study (Kramer & Schmalenburg, 1988), the importance of the role of the first-line manager was stressed. It is also widely acknowledged that the nurse manager is crucial to the delivery of quality patient care and the control of costs (Eubanks, 1992). Unfortunately, there is a sparsity of empirical studies of the nurse manager, especially in view of the importance placed on the role.

Hodges, Knapp, and Cooper (1987) reported the increasing complexity of the practice of the head nurse, and a study by Taunton, Krampitz, and Woods (1989) supported the proposition that the nurse manager is an important factor in retention of professional staff in hospitals. The negative effects of role stress on nurse executives were reported by Scalzi (1988), but data specific to the nurse manager role are needed. Even though research has demonstrated a direct link between nurse autonomy and quality of care (Knaus, Draper, Wagner, & Zimmerman, 1986), and even though dissatisfied nurses can negatively affect patient care and patients' compliance with treatment (Hinshaw, Smeltzer, & Atwood, 1987; Weisman & Nathanson, 1985), studies of this type have not been extended to consider the impact of the nurse manager on quality and patient satisfaction.

ROLE REDESIGN

In 1990, the American Organization of Nurse Executives conducted a national survey to determine the current and predicted roles and responsibilities of nurse managers in health care institutions. Their study (American Organization of Nurse Executives, 1992) offers guidelines for the roles and functions considered integral to the role but does not include information on implementation of the change process. Nurse manager role redesign should be accomplished utilizing basic redesign theory and process.

Role redesign is methodologically similar to any other scientific process. The first step in the redesign process is assessment of existing roles in order to accurately diagnose the need for redesign (Hackman & Oldham, 1980). The second phase is the diagnosis of the problems and the formulation of the goals for the planned change. The second phase follows and depends on the successful completion of Phase 1 (Hackman & Oldham, 1980).

Often, the diagnosis of the need for change is done implicitly or intuitively. However, relying on general perceptions can lead to a flawed diagnosis that leads to inappropriate changes. Thus a systematic assessment is necessary to provide specific data to guide the change process. From the data collected in the assessment phase, the need for and feasibility of role redesign are determined, and specific implementation plans are formulated. The final phase in the redesign process is the evaluation phase. Baseline data from the initial assessment are used to evaluate the results achieved in terms of the goals that were formulated for the specific organization.

Unfortunately, many redesign projects in nursing are implemented without benefit of an organized empirical process. The rate of change in organizations demands a rapid response to the need for new professional roles, yet it is imperative that redesign progress in an orderly manner and produce empirical data to guide future change. Therefore, the purpose of this chapter is to present the rationale, methodology, and results of nurse manager role redesign in an acute care setting.

THEORETICAL FRAMEWORK

An integration of concepts from sociotechnical systems theory, role theory, and job characteristics theory provided the conceptual basis for this research on the head nurse role at the organizational subunit level of analysis. A sociotechnical system is any unit in the organization composed of a technological and a social subsystem having a common task or goal. The organizational subunit is the point of interface between society and the organization. The goals and values of the institution are communicated from top administration to the client through the interface at the unit level.

Role theory provides a set of concepts and relationships for predicting performance in a given role, and has provided a useful framework for the study of nursing roles for the past 20 years. Role conflict, role ambiguity, and role deprivation have been found to be negatively related to nursing job satisfaction, registered nurse retention, and quality of care, and to negatively affect performance in many specialties and at every level of the nursing hierarchy (Lambert & Lambert, 1988; Tumulty, 1992b).

Job characteristics, including both objective and perceptual dimensions of task-related activities, are related to job satisfaction and performance (Hackman & Oldham, 1980). Since its inception, the job characteristics theory has demonstrated its usefulness for job redesign, but there is additional evidence that the model could be enhanced through expansion (Berlinger, Glick, & Rodgers, 1988). Role dynamics may overshadow the specific tasks in jobs of enlarged scope; therefore, combining the most salient role and job characteristics into a role redesign model for nursing appears appropriate.

This theoretical framework was used in the development of the role characteristics model that was previously tested in 10 hospitals and 110 nursing units using a cross-sectional correlational design. Results of the correlation and regression analysis supported the validity of the model. Head nurse role characteristics were found to explain 52% of the variance in head nurse job satisfaction, and were also significantly related to registered nurse retention, patient satisfaction, and quality of care (Tumulty, 1992a). A significant positive relationship between autonomy and patient satisfaction, and between feedback and registered nurse retention, indicated that increasing autonomy and feedback for the head nurse could improve patient satisfaction and registered nurse retention. The job satisfaction of the head nurse explained 17% of the variance in registered nurse retention and seems inconsistent to results described below. Head nurses were particularly unhappy with their workload and with their participation in administrative decisions as well as many other aspects of their role. This initial testing of a model across 10 hospitals also demonstrated significant differences across institutions. More than 50% of the explained variance was at the organizational level. For example, the head nurses in some hospitals perceived more autonomy, received more feedback, had less role conflict, and were significantly more satisfied. The same hospitals where the head nurses were more satisfied achieved the best outcomes in terms of registered nurse retention, patient satisfaction, and quality of care. These results suggest that the redesign of roles in specific organizations could result in greater registered nurse job satisfaction, reduced turnover, and improved quality of care, and that redesign efforts should focus on head nurse as well as staff nurse roles.

THE REDESIGN PROCESS

The first phase of the redesign process at a large metropolitan hospital began in November 1990, when all nursing personnel were asked to complete a compilation of questionnaires distributed to them by the principal investigator. The instruments are described in the next section. This portion of the project was guided by the following research question: Do nurse manager role characteristics change significantly over time following role redesign? Although the redesign process involved the entire nursing department, the focus for this discussion is limited to the nurse manager role.

Collection of Data

Instruments. The instruments used to collect data on the nurse managers were the Index of Work Satisfaction (Stamps & Piedmonte, 1986), the Job Diagnostic Survey (Hackman & Oldham, 1975), the Role Conflict Ambiguity Scale (Rizzo, House, & Lirtzman, 1970), and the Downs-Hazen Scale (Downs & Hazen, 1977). All are well-established and tested instruments with good reported reliability with nursing populations.

The Job Diagnostic Survey (JDS) was developed by Hackman and Oldham (1975) as part of a Yale University study of jobs and how people react to them. The JDS provides a measure of how much autonomy actually exists in the job as perceived by the job incumbent, and consists of 90 items with a 7-point Likert-type scale. Internal consistency reliability of the scale averages .88, and discriminant validity of the items is reported (Hackman & Oldham, 1980).

The JDS described above and the Downs-Hazen Scale provide feedback data. Downs and Hazen (1977) developed an instrument containing eight general factors of communication: personal feedback, corporate perspective, organizational integration, relations with supervisor, relations with subordinates, media quality, horizontal informal communication, and communication climate. In a study of 137 first-line supervisors, Crino and White (1981) supported the validity of the Downs-Hazen scale using factor analysis. Internal consistency for the subscales in that sample, measured by Cronbach's alpha, were .75 to .86, with overall scale reliability of .90.

The Role Conflict/Ambiguity Scale is a 30-item questionnaire developed by Rizzo et al. (1970) to measure role conflict and ambiguity. Subjects respond to each role item, indicating the degree to which the condition exists on a 7-point scale. Factor analysis performed by the instrument developers confirmed two factors of conflict and ambiguity. Kuder-Richardson internal consistency reliabilities with Spearman-Brown corrections resulted in reliability scores of .82 for role conflict and .81 for role ambiguity (Rizzo et al., 1970).

The Index of Work Satisfaction (IWS) (Stamps & Piedmonte, 1986) provides the measure of job satisfaction for nurses. The IWS is a 7-point Likert-type scale that measures the current level of satisfaction for each of six work components: autonomy, interaction, pay, professional status, organizational policies, and task requirements. The IWS was first developed in 1972 and revised in 1978 after trial in seven separate institutions with over 250 subjects. Since then, the instrument has been utilized in over 50 studies of nurses in a variety of settings with sample sizes that range from 22 to 450 subjects. Kendall's tau for the final revision of the scale is .87. Cronbach's alpha is .91 for the 44-item scale, and factor analysis confirmed the validity of the subscales (Stamps & Piedmonte, 1986).

Design

A systematic assessment of the nurse manager role was accomplished using the above instruments. These data were analyzed, and aggregate descriptive data on level of job satisfaction and the other variables were organized by unit. This provided baseline assessment data from which to draw conclusions.

The baseline data were reported to the Nursing Executive Committee, nurse managers, and nursing staff of the hospital. The data revealed low levels of autonomy, feedback, and multiple facets of job satisfaction for all nurses and especially for the 33 responding nurse managers.

Based on these findings, a job redesign and restructuring was undertaken to improve job satisfaction, reduce turnover, and improve performance in order to enhance the quality of patient care and quality of work life for the nurse managers.

A multiple group time series design was chosen to determine changes over time as the redesign progressed. Data were collected prior to and at successive 6-month time periods after implementation of role changes.

Implementation of Role Changes

The decision was made that the role redesign would be based on implementation of primary nursing throughout the hospital, with the goal of redirecting the focus of care to the nurse-patient relationship and providing a foundation for case management. A nationally known nursing consultant was engaged to prepare nurses and nurse managers for the role changes. The education and preparation occurred over a 1-year period. The redesign of the nurse manager role was critical to the redesign project. The limited autonomy in the nurse manager role was seen as an impediment to expanding the autonomy of the staff nurse. A centralized hierarchical structure was also problematic in that it inhibited decision making for both nurse managers and staff nurses (see Figure 3.1). The absence of the nurse manager title from the original organization chart is indicative of the lack of emphasis placed on this role. A decentralization of the nursing department was initiated in conjunction with the role redesign. The department of nursing was reorganized along product lines to clearly delineate the renewed emphasis on the client. The new organizational chart reflects the client emphasis and the decentralization that occurred (see Figure 3.2). Although the number of nurse managers was maintained, the number of clinical directors decreased and the nature of their role changed to allow for more autonomous functioning of the nurse managers.

In conjunction with the structural decentralization, nurse manager role changes were also instituted. One objective was to lessen the clinical emphasis and enhance the managerial aspects of the job. In concert with the objective of driving decision making closer to the customer, the nurse managers were given increased responsibility for the budgeting and personnel management processes and were encouraged to delegate clinical and staffing decisions to the primary nurses. Where, previously, nurse managers had assumed the role of clinical charge nurse for patient care, the role was refocused to include all personnel management issues—hiring, firing, and evaluation as well as preparation and management of their nursing unit budgets—many of which were

(text continued on page 29)

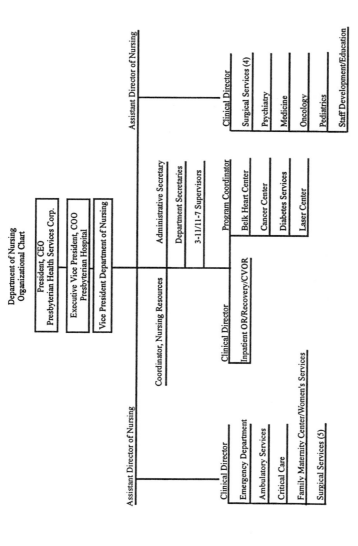

Figure 3.1. Organization of Presbyterian Hospital Department of Nursing Before Restructuring
SOURCE: Reprinted with permission from Department of Nursing, Presbyterian Hospital, Charlotte, NC.

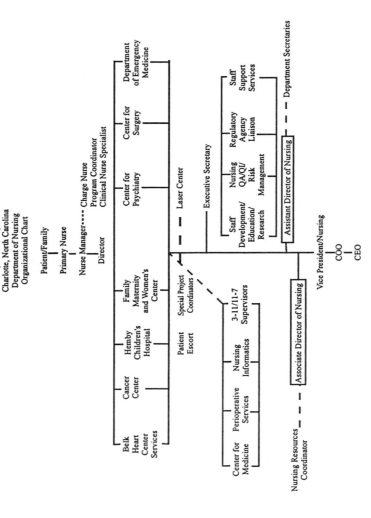

Figure 3.2. Organization of Presbyterian Hospital Department of Nursing After Restructuring

SOURCE: Reprinted with permission from Department of Nursing, Presbyterian Hospital, Charlotte, NC.

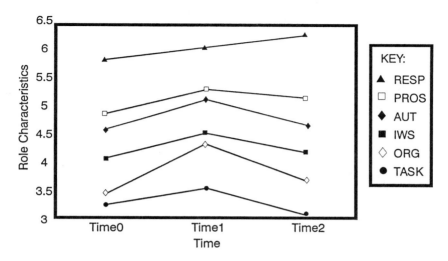

Figure 3.3. Trends in Role Characteristics Over Time Subsequent to Role Redesign

responsibilities previously assumed by the clinical director. This allowed the primary nurses to assume greater responsibility for patient care standards, quality management, and collaboration with other direct caregivers. The literature supports decentralization and role changes of this type to improve retention and satisfaction of staff nurses and improve quality of care for the patients (Hinshaw et al., 1987; Knaus et al., 1986; Kramer & Schmalenburg, 1988).

Results

Initial data from the 33 responding nurse managers (90% of the initial sample) indicated serious role problems in the areas of satisfaction, autonomy, organizational policies, and status. Overall job satisfaction (IWS) was 4.1, with autonomy (AUT) only slightly better at 4.5 (see Figure 3.3). Satisfaction with organizational policies (ORG) was only 3.5, $SD = 1.1$; satisfaction with tasks (TASK) was 3.23, $SD = .81$; professional status (PROF) was 4.85, $SD = .74$; and responsibility for the work (RESP) was somewhat higher at 5.8, $SD = .56$. Because these concepts were all measured on a 7-point Likert-type scale, none were in the positive range except responsibility for work. Other study variables reflected the same pattern of low to neutral responses. Even conflict and ambiguity were relatively low, indicating that although the nurse managers were not particularly satisfied, they were also not experiencing a great deal of role stress.

TABLE 3.1   The Effects of Role Redesign on Nurse Manager Satisfaction With
            Organizational Policies

Source	df	SS	MS	F	p
Between groups	2	11.9	5.9	5.1	.008*
Within groups	75	88.3	1.1		
Total	77	100.3			

*$p < .05$.

The restructuring and role changes described above were implemented
during 1991, and in the spring of 1992 and again in the fall of 1992 (6 months
later) the nurse managers were resurveyed. The trends for the above variables
are shown in Figure 3.3. As can be clearly seen, there was a fairly dramatic improvement in satisfaction with the role characteristics from Time 0 (baseline)
to Time 1. The changes from Time 1 to Time 2 are less dramatic and show a
regression toward the baseline. All of the variables under study showed similar
trends. An analysis of variance demonstrated significant changes over time for
only two of the variables: organizational policies and responsibility for work
(see Tables 3.1 and 3.2). The Sheffé Multiple Range Test was performed and
revealed a significant change at Time 1 for organizational policies and at Time
2 for responsibility for work. No other variables in the study changed significantly over time, but all showed a trend in the positive direction.

Discussion

This study confirms that positive changes in the quality of work life for the
nurse manager can be achieved through role redesign. The nurse managers in
this study perceived the organizational policies significantly more positively
than they did previously. This improvement in hospital policies may also have
contributed to the subsequent changes in other feelings of job satisfaction. The
nurse managers also felt significantly more responsibility for their work. This
can only lead to increased positive outcomes for the hospital.

The results reported here also remind us that role changes develop slowly
over time and need to be studied accordingly. The initial excitement of the
change project may simulate a Hawthorne effect, and initial positive results
need to be interpreted with this in mind. Much more important to the health
care environment is the maintenance of sustained positive changes over time.
An advantage of a time series design is the usefulness of the data in guiding the
redesign process. The data can be immediately utilized by the nurse executive
to evaluate and, if necessary, redirect the redesign process. In this instance, an
attempt is being made to ensure that role changes are maintained and insti-

TABLE 3.2 The Effects of Role Redesign on Nurse Manager Responsibility for Work

Source	df	SS	MS	F	p
Between groups	2	2.2	1.1	4.1	.008*
Within groups	76	20.6	.3		
Total	78	22.83			

*$p < .05$.

tutionalized. Additional data collection is also planned to ensure that trends continue in the desired direction. Carefully designed studies to capture the effects of changes over time are an essential part of a successful redesign project. In this instance, the positive results already achieved for the nurse managers, and those anticipated in the future, can contribute significantly to the success of the organization.

REFERENCES

American Organization of Nurse Executives. (1992). The role and functions of the hospital nurse manager. *Nursing Management, 23*(9), 36-38.

Berlinger, L., Glick, W., & Rodgers, R. (1988). Job enrichment and performance improvement. In J. Campbell & R. Campbell (Eds.), *Productivity in organizations: New perspectives from industrial and organizational psychology* (pp. 219-254). San Francisco: Jossey-Bass.

Crino, M., & White, M. (1981). Satisfaction in communication: An examination of the Downs-Hazen Measure. *Psychological Reports, 49,* 831-838.

Downs, C., & Hazen, M. (1977). A factor analytic study of communication satisfaction. *Journal of Business Communication, 14,* 63-73.

Eubanks, P. (1992). The new nurse manager: A linchpin in quality care and cost control. *Hospitals, 66*(8) 22-30.

Hackman, R., & Oldham, G. (1975). Development of the Job Diagnostic Survey. *Journal of Applied Psychology, 60*(2), 159-170.

Hackman, R., & Oldham, G. (1980). *Work redesign.* Reading, MA: Addison-Wesley.

Hinshaw, A., Smeltzer, C., & Atwood, J. (1987). Innovative retention strategies for nursing staff. *Journal of Nursing Administration, 17*(4), 12-20.

Hodges, L., Knapp, R., & Cooper, J. (1987). Innovative retention strategies for nursing staff. *Journal of Nursing Administration, 17*(6), 8-16.

Knaus, W., Draper, E., Wagner, D., & Zimmerman, J. (1986). An evaluation of outcomes from intensive care in major medical centers. *Annals of Internal Medicine, 10,* 410-418.

Kramer, M., & Schmalenburg, C. (1988). Magnet hospital: Part II—Institutions of excellence. *Journal of Nursing Administration, 18*(2), 11-18.

Lambert, C., & Lambert, V. (1988). A review and synthesis of the research on role conflict and its impact on nurses involved in faculty practice programs. *Journal of Nursing Education, 27,* 54-60.

McClure, M., Poulin, M., Sovie, M., & Wandelt, M. (1983). *Magnet hospitals: Attraction and retention of professional nurses.* Kansas City, MO: American Nurses Association.

Moritz, P., Hinshaw, A., & Heinrich, J. (1989). Nursing resources and the delivery of patient care: The National Center for Nursing Research perspective. *Journal of Nursing Administration, 19,* 12-18.

Rizzo, J., House, R., & Lirtzman, S. (1970). Role conflict and ambiguity in complex organizations. *Administrative Science Quarterly, 15*, 150-163.

Scalzi, C. (1988). Role stress and coping strategies of nurse executives. *Journal of Nursing Administration, 18*(3), 34-37.

Stamps, P., & Piedmonte, E. (1986). *Nurses and work satisfaction.* Lexington, MA: D. C. Heath.

Taunton, R., Krampitz, S., & Woods, C. (1989). Manager impact on retention of hospital staff: Part 1. *Journal of Nursing Administration, 19*(3), 7-18.

Tumulty, G. (1992a). Head nurse role redesign: Improving satisfaction and performance. *Journal of Nursing Administration, 22*,(2), 41-47.

Tumulty, G. (1992b). A model for nursing role redesign. In B. Henry (Ed.), *Practice and inquiry for nursing administration* (pp. 67-71). Washington, DC: American Academy of Nursing.

Weisman, C., & Nathanson, C. (1985). Professional satisfaction and client outcomes. *Medical Care, 23*, 1179-1191.

CHAPTER 4

Multiple Productivity Evaluation to Support Nursing System Redesign

Carol A. Brooks
Paul E. Juras

Evaluation methods that provide information on technology and structural characteristics associated with efficient systems are essential to the meaningful redesign of nursing care delivery systems. This chapter reports on an investigation of an approach known as data envelopment analysis for determining relative technical efficiency of nursing units. Relationships of efficiency ratings to specific delivery systems' technological and structural characteristics are then reported in order to identify characteristics associated with the rating of nursing unit efficiency.

Evaluation methods that provide information on combinations of technological and structural characteristics associated with efficient systems are essential for the meaningful restructuring of nursing care delivery systems. Lack of consensus on methodology for measuring multivariate systems' efficiency has resulted both from and in data collection and analysis that are insufficient for adequate evaluation purposes. Multivariate evaluation methods designed to monitor both clinical outcomes of care and the inputs (resources in time and dollars) required to achieve the desired outcomes are the tools needed to provide data for meaningful restructuring of nursing care delivery systems. Meaningful restructuring means organizing and evaluating work around costs and outcomes, not discrete tasks such as nursing care planning or scheduling. Analysis of critical measures of performance, such as cost, quality, service, and speed, is fundamental to the rethinking and radical redesign of nursing systems that is essential for the dramatic improvements needed.

A postulate of organizational literature is that the proper fit between technology and structure on work units is imperative for these units to operate efficiently and effectively (Child, 1972; Perrow, 1967; Woodward, 1965). A model has been developed to suggest appropriate fits between technological and structural dimensions on nursing units (Alexander & Bauerschmidt, 1987). *Technology for nursing units* is defined as the acts performed by nursing personnel to change the status of an individual from a patient to a discharged person, and *structure* is defined as the allocation of work roles and administrative mechanisms to control work activities (Alexander & Bauerschmidt, 1987). To develop a structural contingency model that is prescriptive and theoretical, evaluation methods for testing the model are essential.

Utilizing a production equation with nurse expert agreed-upon inputs and outputs that represent both qualitative and quantitative values provides a method for obtaining technical efficiency ratings for multivariate comparable systems. Relative and technical efficiency measures the ability to convert units of input into units of output. The efficiency ratio then is capable of serving as a dependent variable in regression equations that use structural and technological characteristics of systems as independent variables to determine ratios.

This chapter reports on a two-phase evaluation study carried out on 41 medical units in 21 selected New York State hospitals. The first phase of the study was designed to investigate utilization of data envelopment analysis (DEA) for multiple variable management in determining the relative technical efficiency of the selected units. DEA, an approach to multiple productivity measures, is a form of linear programming developed by Charnes and Cooper (1985) that is a useful method for determining the relative efficiency of units with multiple inputs and outputs. The second phase was designed to determine the association of specific structural and technological characteristics with the relative efficiency ratings of the nursing units studied.

Major concepts relative to the study are technical and relative efficiency, data envelopment analysis, and inputs and outputs.

TECHNICAL AND RELATIVE EFFICIENCY

A traditional engineering concept of efficiency compares actual output to optimal output for a given input or set of inputs. If the quantity of each input required and the substitutability of inputs are known, the identification of a technical production function is possible. Unfortunately, despite the efforts of Feldstein (1968) and others (e.g., Dowling, 1976), a generally accepted production function for nursing units does not exist in either physical or financial terms (Berki, 1972).

Anthony and Young (1988) pointed out that dealing with multiple inputs and outputs simultaneously reduces the ability to develop engineering standards. Nunamaker (1983) suggested that the use of a reference set of hospitals to measure efficiency is a desirable course of action. This was the course of action followed in this study. An objective of the first phase of the study was to identify the production function that was technically best, given the boundaries that exist, to determine relative technical efficiency.

Relative efficiency is a concept proposed by Farrell (1957). If an organization has relative efficiency, it cannot produce the same output with fewer inputs or produce more outputs with the same inputs. This concept "assumes that a reduction in any input or an expansion in any output has some value and does not require that these values be stipulated in any way" (Charnes, Cooper, & Rhodes, 1978, p. 433).

Technical efficiency, on the other hand, stipulates that there is a maximum level of output for any combination of inputs, but there is no minimal output level, which allows for technical inefficiency to exist. The technically efficient production function is not necessarily optimum, for the "wrong" set of inputs may be used in a technically efficient manner. This condition is possible because there are multiple production functions for any given level of output. An example is reports of outputs of high levels of client and staff satisfaction produced by systems using varied roles and functions for different levels of nursing staff. The result is that technical efficiency is not equal to economic efficiency (Berki, 1972).

The distinction between economic and technical efficiency is important because the resources available determine which production functions are feasible (Berki, 1972). It is also possible that a set of feasible production functions will not contain a theoretical economic optimum. The stipulation of theoretical economic optimums for nursing production functions of diagnosing and treating humans' responses to optimizing their health status is a well-recognized dilemma. Also, types of available inputs and costs of inputs differ from one setting to another. The result is that two identical nursing production units might have different economically efficient production functions solely due to the different types of inputs and the cost differential of the units.

The ideal input to a given production function or technology may not be available, at least in the short term. The best a nursing department can do is use its available resources (inputs) most efficiently (technical efficiency). "In effect we are concerned not with planning a production unit, but with the operation of an existing one" (Berki, 1972, p. 51). Data envelopment analysis (DEA) provides a means of measuring relative efficiency and determining technical efficiency.

DATA ENVELOPMENT ANALYSIS

Data envelopment analysis is a linear programming (LP) approach that depends upon creating a relatively efficient unit from a combination of other units' inputs and outputs (Banker & Morey, 1986). Units are referred to as *decision-making units* (DMUs). Units are then evaluated against the artificially created composite unit. The level of efficiency is valued in direct proportion to the distance of the observed point from the *frontier production function,* the production function that minimizes the quality of resources (inputs) used for a given level of outputs (see Figure 4.1).

In a single-output, two-input situation, a production function would be:

$$Y = F(x_1, x_2)$$

where Y is output and is a function of inputs x_1 and x_2.

In Figure 4.1, the output Y of each unit j is divided into the respective quantities of inputs x_1 and x_2. Point a represents an observed value for a unit not on the efficient frontier. Point A is the composite DMU against which observed DMU A is evaluated. The level of inefficiency is valued in direct proportion to the distance of the observed from the frontier, which in this illustration is the value of Oa/OA.

Note that DEA uses a piecemeal linear approach. Any observed point will be compared to the facet (linear segment) intersected by the ray drawn from the origin (O) to the observed point. Any standard linear programming package can be used to solve the formulation.[1]

The DEA technique is an attempt to determine the degree to which a unit converts its inputs to outputs, without waste, relative to its peers. The efficiency score relates to efficiency according to a proportionate contraction of resources criteria (Nunamaker, 1983). Those units that receive a score of 1 when using the weights derived for the created DMU make up the reference set. When a unit receives a score of less than 1, "the DEA results will indicate which resources are being over-utilized and which outputs are being overproduced" (Sexton et al., 1989, p. 154).

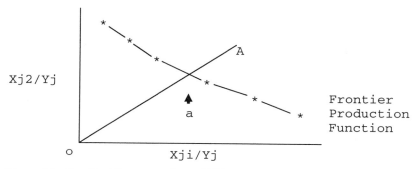

Figure 4.1. Graphical Representation of DEA

Use of other techniques to identify an efficient unit production function has been rejected for several reasons. Econometric regression techniques estimate central tendencies. Translog analysis yields estimates of average production functions but is not as flexible in approximating true production functions (Banker, Charnes, Cooper, & Mainderatta, 1987). Ratio analysis limits analysis to a single user input/output relationship.

Estimating a nursing unit function by assuming a parametric form is difficult because of the multiple inputs and outputs. This difficulty is compounded by the absence of a market to determine values for many of the nursing unit outputs, such as patient knowledge and skill necessary for discharge, and some of the inputs, such as patient's level of wellness. DEA provides a nonparametrical mathematical programming technique for evaluating the relative productivity of the nursing units, thus avoiding the problems of imposing a particular functional form.

Limitations of DEA

The DEA technique is not designed to identify the optimal production function. Because all nursing units under study may have one or more inefficiencies of operation, not all the inefficient units may be identified. This result may occur because DEA is limited to identifying a relatively efficient production function from the reported data. However, this study was only designed to determine which characteristics of the units in the study group were associated with more efficient use of resources.

Sexton (1989) noted that the efficiency measure of any DMU is expressed in terms of relativity to the set of DMUs being evaluated. As a result, changes in the study set are likely to change the efficiency scores. Epstein and Henderson (1989) also noted that efficiency scores are monotonically nonincreasing with respect to the addition of DMUs because each DMU adds a new constraint to the linear programming problem. A rule of thumb is to have a study group at least three times as large as the combined number of inputs and outputs (Banker, Charnes, Cooper, Swarts, & Thomas, 1989). The sample size of this study was sufficient to meet this heuristic.

There are aspects of efficiency that DEA does not address. For example, price efficiency, the practice of buying the lowest cost supplies or services, might be evaluated through the use of ratio analysis such as cost per full-time equivalent or cost per supply unit.

The critical steps in the application of DEA are identification of candidate variables, variable selection, and variable measurement (Epstein & Henderson, 1989). Because DEA has a free functional form, no restrictions are placed on the production relationship, which only assumes convexity and linearity. Each variable included has an equal opportunity to influence efficiency; thus variable selection is critical.

Managerial Use of DEA

DEA results lead "to highly specific managerial strategies for improving the efficiency of an inefficient DMU by indicating which inputs are being under-produced and in each case by how much" (Sexton et al., 1989, p. 1187). Sexton et al. (1989, p. 1176) showed that "DEA can provide useful information that highlights for managers how their programs and facilities can absorb pending budget cuts without affecting service delivery."

Huang and McLaughlin (1989) made use of DEA to identify the sources and amount of inefficiency in rural health centers in North Carolina. Banker et al. (1989) used DEA specifically to develop cost standards for departments (but not individual nursing units) in a number of hospitals.

The purpose of system redesign is to increase the efficiency of resource utilization. With efficient resource utilization as the objective, it is reasonable to use this objective as a basis of performance evaluation. In the absence of an ideal level of production that can be used for evaluation, peer comparison is offered as an alternative (Nunamaker, 1983). A measure of relative efficiency is selected because of the lack of an agreed-upon comprehensive production function for nursing units.

Lewin and Minton (1986) stated that it would be desirable to have a theory-based technique for calculating the relative efficiency of an organization (either over time or in comparison to other referent organizations) that would be

1. Capable of identifying the most efficient organizations relative to others
2. Capable of deriving a single measure of relative efficiency in terms of resource utilization

3. Not dependent upon a priori weights
4. Able to handle qualitative factors
5. Able to provide insight as to factors that contribute to relative efficiency

DEA meets these requirements. The selection and measurement of inputs and outputs to be used as variables were major considerations in the proper application of this efficiency measurement tool.

INPUTS AND OUTPUTS

The objective was to select a set of inputs and outputs that would be relevant from a technical efficiency perspective. Input and output data were collected for the period January 1 to March 30, 1990. Inputs were broken down into three groups: (a) labor, (b) capital, and (c) materials and other. The first input was labor hours by level of personnel, which was broken down into three groups: (a) unit management, (b) internal staff, including per diem and float personnel, and (c) outside agency staff. *Capital* was defined as open beds on the unit. Measures of material and other inputs selected were volume of laboratory tests, radiology procedures, and number of medications. Because few nursing departments were able to provide the material data broken down by unit, these measures could not be used in this study. Table 4.1 contains a list of the input measures used.

The ideal output would be a measure of whether expected changes in health status were obtained. This approach would require a case-by-case analysis of each patient, giving consideration to age, preexisting conditions, health history, severity of illness, and diagnosis. It would also require the development of a generally accepted index of health status. These are unreasonable expectations at the present time, but worthy of future consideration as nursing data sets and informatics are developed.

Patient days was selected as the best available measure of resource utilization. A major indicator of a hospital's financial performance and predictor of resource consumption in the system is the patient's length of stay (LOS) (Joel, 1984; Shaffer, 1983). Even if two different nursing units produce the same relative mix of outputs for the same quantity of inputs, differences in quality may still produce differences in technical efficiency.

The first selected indicator of quality was the occurrence of infections acquired during the hospital stay (nosocomial infections). Prevention of complications is a goal of nursing care, and infections are examples of complications that increase a patient's LOS (Lowenstein, 1989). Haley, White, Culver, and Hughes (1987) found that more than 95% of cost savings from preventing infections translate into financial gain for a hospital.

TABLE 4.1 Input Measures

Name	Definition
HEAD	Head nurse hours worked
RN	RN hours worked, including per diem and float hours worked
LPN	LPN hours worked, including per diem and float hours worked
AIDE	Nurse aide hours worked, including per diem and float hours worked
OTHR	Other staff hours worked, including per diem and float hours worked
RN_OUT	RN external agency personnel hours worked
LPN_OUT	LPN external agency personal hours worked
AIDE_OUT	Nurse aide external agency hours worked
OPEN_BED	Number of open beds

TABLE 4.2 Output Measures

Name	Definition
PAT_DAYS	Number of patient days. This is calculated by multiplying the number of patients treated by the average length of stay.
NO_FALLS	Patients treated minus number of patient falls
NO_INFEC	Patients treated minus number of infections
NO_INCID	Patients treated minus (reportable incidents minus number of reportable falls)
PATIENTS TREATED	Number of admissions to the study unit plus the number of patients transferred to the unit

The second quality indicator was the number of patient falls. Falls may result in the patient's needing additional treatment, thereby increasing costs and potentially increasing the length of stay.

A final quality indicator was reportable incidents. A reportable incident is any incident that may prolong a patient's length of stay. Such incidents must be reported to the state health department in New York State. Table 4.2 provides a summary of all the outputs used in the first phase of the study.

SAMPLE

The 1990 list of members of the American Organization of Nurse Executives was used to identify individuals in New York State hospitals to contact for participation in this study. Only those executives from New York State hospitals that have medical units were contacted. Seventy-five nurse executives were identified and asked to participate in the study.

TABLE 4.3 Characteristics of Participants

Characteristic	Respondents[a]
Bed size	
High	1,184
Low	54
Average	387
Occupancy percentage	
High	92.2
Low	64.8
Average	80.9
Teaching status	
Teaching	12
Nonteaching	10

a. $N = 22$; includes the hospital for which the data were subsequently dropped.

Forty-two (56%) of the nurse executives contacted indicated an interest in participating in the study. Of the original 42 people indicating an interest in the study, 22 (52%) actually provided data.

One of the hospitals that provided data was dropped because the data were for the wrong time period. The net result was that usable data were collected from 21 hospitals representing a total of 41 nursing units. Information about the participants is contained in Table 4.3.

EFFICIENCY DETERMINATION

The main objective of Phase 1 was to use DEA to determine a relative efficiency measure of each nursing unit. Because this was an exploratory study, a number of combinations of inputs and outputs (runs) were used. Nunamaker (1983) suggested that DEA's usefulness would be improved if it were used to calculate efficiency scores using a variety of sets. Twelve different calculations of efficiency were conducted. Primary decisions on set selection related to the level to which labor data were to be disaggregated and how best to use the capital measure of beds.

Labor disaggregation issues related to attempts to lump together RNs having overall leadership/management responsibilities and no responsibilities for individual nursing care of patients with RNs having responsibility for individual nursing care of patients. Runs combining assistant head nurse hours with staff hours and with head nurse hours were carried out. The two groupings showed no differences in effects on efficiency, as shown by Pearson and Spearman coefficients calculated. The other issues dealt with were whether to combine float and per diem hours with unit-specific staff and whether to combine external agency staff hours with employed staff hours or deal with them separately. These issues were identified because of generalized assumptions that have been made regarding inefficiencies produced by staff working on units to which they are not routinely assigned. Comparing runs using different combinations of these resources through use of Spearman tests and Pearson correlation coefficients showed strong correlations with no noteworthy effects on the efficiency ratings.

Runs were conducted using occupied beds as a measure of capital and open beds. This was done for two reasons: (a) There is a general feeling expressed in the industry that occupancy does not reflect adequately the use of capital, and (b) because occupancy rates were so high (an average of 90.4%), there was interest in determining if the different measures would have different effects on the efficiency ratings. A Friedman rank test was used to determine whether the measure of capital used caused changes in the ranked efficiency scores of the nursing units. Because there were three different labor combinations and one different output combination, the Friedman test was repeated four times.

The null hypothesis for each test was

H_0: The efficiency rankings of the nursing units are equally likely.

The null for each test was rejected at the .99 level. The results indicated that the type of capital measure included as an input had little effect on efficiency for data used in this study.

Interpretation of a Sample DEA Report

Table 4.4 is part of a DEA report. The report is for DMU #10, which had an efficiency score of .6399, meaning that a composite DMU could be formed that would provide the same level of output as DMU #10 but use substantially less inputs; the composite DMU would contain some of the characteristics of DMUs #5 and #21, as indicated by their inclusion as facet members.

The column labeled "Value If Efficient" shows the amount of each input that would have been used if DMU #10 had been efficient. The weights (lambda values) indicate that DMU #10 should try to emulate DMU #5 more than DMU #21. The slack values indicate amounts of inefficiencies. They indicate that although the unit was making good use of the RN staff (RN & Asst), it was also using per diem and float RNs (RN D & F) that were apparently not needed. The slack values indicate a potential to reduce the level of non-RN staff in the unit. There were no other units from the same hospital, so it was not possible

TABLE 4.4 Sample DEA Report

	DECISION-MAKING UNIT #10 (hospital 120 unit A) EFFICIENCY SCORE = .6399		
	FACET: LAMBDA =	5 .942	21 .058
INPUTS	(A) ACTUAL VALUE	(B) VALUE IF EFFICIENT	(A-B) SLACK
HEAD	672.0	371.6	300.4
RN+ASST	5937.9	5876.8	61.4
LPN_WK	4312.1	1422.9	2889.2
AIDE_WK	2944.8	1187.1	1757.7
OTHER_WK	2203.5	864.9	1338.6
RN_D&F	396.0	.0	396.0
LPN_D&F	6.0	.0	6.0
AIDE_D&F	240.0	.0	240.0
OTHR_D&F	60.0	.0	60.0
RN_OUT	.0	.0	.0
LPN_OUT	.0	.0	.0
AIDE_OUT	.0	.0	.0
OPEN_BED	31.0	28.1	2.9

NOTE: The variables are defined in Table 4.1.

to determine whether some hospital-wide factors were causing the inefficiency. This example is provided to illustrate how sources and amounts of inefficiency can be identified.

RESULTS OF FIRST PHASE

The results of the first phase of the analysis indicated that 13 of the 41 units (32%) were relatively inefficient. The efficiency scores of the inefficient units ranged from .51 to .86. Due to the nature of the inefficiency measure, tests of the statistical significance of the scores were not performed. The second phase of the analysis examined the level of association between selected hospital-wide and nursing structural and technological characteristics and the efficiency ratings of the nursing units.

Relationship of Nursing Unit Characteristics to Efficiency Ratings

Specific items addressed were use of unit dose medication systems, use of computerized documentation systems, presence of a unit management program, use of rotating shifts, nursing staff performance of housekeeping duties, use of acuity data to prepare staff budget, and provision of data that compare actual and required nursing care hours. Structural and technological characteristics selected were based on input from nursing management and staff as to characteristics that negatively or positively influenced their efficiency.

This portion of the analysis was done in two steps. The first step was to use the Mann-Whitney test to determine if there was a statistical difference in the distribution of the ranks of the efficiency score of those units with a specific characteristic versus those without the characteristic. The null hypothesis in each case was stated in the following manner:

H_0: There is no difference in the distribution of ranks of the nursing units that have the selected characteristic compared to those without the characteristic.

The test described above was conducted in conjunction with regression analysis to determine if there was consistency in the findings.

The DEA results served as the dependent variable, and the different operating characteristics and management techniques served as the independent variables to the stepwise forward selection process used for the regression analysis. The criterion for entry was that the coefficient of the characteristic had to have a p value of $\leq .25$.

Only three of the unit-specific characteristics were found to be statistically associated with relative technical efficiency: the use of rotating shifts (negative association), the use of acuity data to prepare the staff budget (positive association), and the use of computerized documentation (negative association).

Relationship of Structural and Technological Characteristics to Efficiency Ratings

All of the characteristics discussed up to this point are nursing-unit-specific characteristics. In other words, not all units in the same hospital will necessarily have these same characteristics. However, hospital-wide characteristics, most notably teaching status, may have an effect on nursing unit efficiency.

One cannot be sure that teaching status has a hospital-wide effect or a specific effect on certain areas within the hospitals. It is commonly believed that teaching hospitals treat the most severe patients because these hospitals are likely to be the most advanced in their methods of treatment. Because this determination is an unresolved empirical issue, teaching hospitals were included in the study. If the units in these types of hospitals turned out to be consistently less efficient than their nonteaching counterparts, the nursing units in the teaching hospitals would have to be analyzed separately.

The second hospital-wide characteristic included was whether the nursing staff was unionized. Because unionization can limit the flexibility of administration in terms of employment practices, nursing unit efficiency may be affected.

The results of the analysis that focused on the hospital-wide characteristics revealed that neither characteristic had a statistically significant regression coefficient. As a result, these characteristics were not controlled for in the analysis of the unit-specific characteristics.

PROBLEMS

Conducting this study revealed that hospital information systems do not seem to support data requests that may come from nursing unit managers. In particular, medication and lab test data are normally tracked at the patient level, not at the unit level. As a result, it was not feasible for all the hospitals to determine which services were provided to patients while they were in specific nursing units.

Prior studies have found that costs vary positively with the number of patients and their severity levels (case mix) (Evans, 1971; Feldstein, 1965; Lave, Lave, & Silverman, 1972). By grouping patients by specific diagnoses, outputs could have been measured as the number of patients treated within each diagnostic group. In effect, a multiproduct definition of output that gives recognition to the number of each type of case treated was needed.

Diagnosis-related groups (DRGs) were to be used as the primary determinant of hospital output because they are an operational output of the prospective pricing system (Cromwell & Pope, 1989). With DRGs as a consistent measure across units and between hospitals, any measure of productivity would have lent itself to comparability across units and among hospitals. Both Nunamaker (1983) and Sherman (1984) indicated that the use of DRGs may have provided more valuable results, and Banker, Conrad, and Strauss (1986) suggested that the use of DRGs would have improved their study. At the same time, Lowenstein (1989) made note of the fact that DRGs are being used to identify nursing costs and assist in the development of new care delivery methods. Although DRG data is collected by the hospital, unit-specific data proved to be generally unavailable. Unit-specific DRG data and a uniform nursing data set would improve the validity, comparability, and collectibility of the data.

RECOMMENDATIONS

*Low productivity may be due to the lack of management attention to
providing a setting which encourages efficient performance.*
(Leher, 1983)

Young and Saltman (1983) pointed out that hospital administrators have
focused their cost-control efforts on the price of inputs rather than the efficiency with which inputs are used. They stated that this condition was due to
the lack of standards for measuring input efficiency. An alternative explanation
is that there is a lack of an adequate information system to provide the necessary
data to measure efficiency. One nurse administrator commented that she is
given a guideline figure for her total budget and told not to exceed that figure.
1991 was the first year she was given information on projected patient census
to prepare her budget. Along these lines, nine respondents (19%) indicated
that data comparing actual to required hours of care were not available to them.

A number of the nursing administrators who participated expressed appreciation for this research effort because it made them aware of types of data they
might find useful. For example, whereas 28 of the 41 nursing units reported
that acuity data were used to plan the staff budget, 13 said that the data were
not used. This raises an important question as to whether these individuals are
aware of the potential benefit of using such data. This reinforces the already
recognized need for education on management decision making.

Nursing management needs to be provided support for the performance
measurement system, including the production process itself. An interesting
finding was that many hospitals do not collect the requested information at the
nursing unit level. Because the nursing units represent the points at which all
the other medical support services come together, this observation is disturb-
ing. This finding echoes the words of Glandon, Colbert, and Thomasma (1989,
p. 30), who wrote, "Nursing executives faced with making difficult operating
decisions often do not have reliable information."

This study also found that the data requested are not collected in a manner
that makes them easily retrievable. The difficulty in retrieving data was reported by five nurse executives as a reason for nonparticipation. However,
there is a growing movement to classify nursing units as profit centers. If this
movement is to be successful, greater attention needs to be focused on the
information needs of nursing unit managers. Development of the hospital
information system needs to be a cooperative effort involving all those who are
affected by it.

The study did not accomplish all that the authors had intended. This failure is due to the deficiencies in the data provided. The inadequacy of the data reinforces the need for improvements in hospital information systems, especially in the area of support for nursing administrators.

Synthesis of nursing and management knowledge is essential to meaningful redesign of nursing systems. To achieve the potential offered by management and nursing colleges' collaboration, further endeavors such as the one described are necessary. Understanding of nursing organizational systems and management knowledge of accounting were essential elements in designing this study to test a method of evaluating the productivity efficiency of nursing units.

NOTE

1. DEA software obtained from the Center for Cybernetic Studies at the University of Texas in Austin was used.

REFERENCES

Alexander, J. W., & Bauerschmidt, A. D. (1987). Implications for nursing administration of the relationship of technology and structure to quality of care. *Nursing Administration Quarterly, 11*(4), 1-10.

Anthony, R. N., & Young, D. W. (1988). *Management control in nonprofit organizations.* Homewood, IL: Irwin.

Banker, R. D. Charnes, A., Cooper, W. W., & Mainderatta, A. (1987). A comparison of DEA and translog estimates of production frontiers using simulated observations from a known technology. In A. Dogramac & R. Fare (Eds.), *Applications of modern production theory: Efficiency and productivity* (pp. 33-55). Boston: Kluwer.

Banker, R. D., Charnes, A., Cooper, W. W., Swarts, J., & Thomas, D. A. (1989). An introduction to data envelopment analysis with some of its models and their uses. In J. L. Chan & J. M. Patton (Eds.), *Research in governmental and nonprofit accounting* (Vol. 5, pp. 125-163). Greenwich, CT: JAI.

Banker, R. D., Conrad, R. F., & Strauss, R. P. (1986). A comparative application of data envelopment analysis and translog methods: An illustration study of hospital production. *Management Science, 32,* 30-44.

Banker, R. D., & Morey, R. C. (1986). Use of categorical variables in data envelopment analysis. *Management Science, 32*(1), 1013-1027.

Berki, S. E. (1972). *Hospital economics.* Lexington, MA: Lexington.

Charnes, A., & Cooper, W. W. (1985). Preface to topics in data envelopment analysis. *Annals of Operation Research, 2,* 59-94.

Charnes, A., Cooper, W. W., & Rhodes, E. (1978). Measuring efficiency of decision making units. *European Journal of Operational Research, 2*(6), 429-444.

Child, J. (1972). Organizational structure, environment and performance: The role of strategic choice. *Sociology, 6*(1), 1-22.

Cromwell, J., & Pope, G. C. (1989). Trends in hospital labor and total factor productivity, 1981-86. *Health Care Financing Review, 10*(4), 39-50.

Dowling, W. L. (1976). *Hospital production.* Lexington MA: Lexington.

Epstein, M. K., & Henderson, F. C. (1989). Data envelopment analysis for managerial control and diagnosis. *Decision Science, 20,* 90-119.

Evans, R. G. (1971, February). Behavioral cost funtions for hospitals. *Canadian Journal of Economics, 4,* 198-215.

Farrell, M. J. (1957). The measurement of productive efficiency. *Canadian Journal of Economics, 20,* 253-290.

Feldstein, M. (1965). Hospital cost variations and case mix differences. *Medical Care, 3,* 95-103.

Feldstein, M. J. (1968). *Economic analysis for health service efficiency.* Amsterdam: North Holland.

Glandon, G. L., Colbert, K. W., & Thomasma, M. (1989, May). Nursing delivery models and RN mix: Cost implications. *Nursing Management, 20*(5), 30-33.

Haley, R. W., White, J. W., Culver, D. H., & Hughes, J. M. (1987). The financial incentive for hospitals to prevent nosocomial infections under the prospective payment system. *Journal of the American Medical Association, 257*(12), 1611-1614.

Huang, Y. G., & McLaughlin, C. P. (1989). Relative efficiency in rural primary health care: An application of data envelopment analysis. *Health Services Research, 24*(2), 143-158.

Joel, L. (1984). DRGs and RIMS: Implications for nursing. *Nursing Outlook, 32*(1), 42-49.

Lave, J. R., Lave, L. B., & Silverman, L. P. (1972). Hospital cost estimation controlling for case mix. *Applied Economics, 4,* 165-180.

Leher, R. N. (1983). *White collar productivity.* New York: McGraw-Hill.

Lewin, A. Y., & Minton, J. W. (1986). Determining organizational effectiveness: Another look, and an agenda for research. *Management Science, 32*(5), 514-538.

Lowenstein, A. (1989). Diagnosis related groups: Controlling health care costs. In C. E. Lambert, Jr., & V. A. Lambert (Eds.), *Perspectives in nursing* (pp. 333-354). Norwalk, CT: Appleton & Lange.

Nunamaker, T. R. (1983). Measuring routine nursing service efficiency: A comparison of cost per patient day and data envelopment analysis models. *Health Services Research, 18*(2), 183-205.

Perrow, C. (1967). A framework for the comparative analysis of organizations. *American Sociological Review, 32*(2), 247-259.

Sexton, T. (1989). The methodology of data envelopment analysis. In R. H. Silkman (Ed.), *Measuring efficiency: An assessment of data envelopment analysis* (pp. 7-23). San Francisco: Jossey-Bass.

Sexton, T. R., Leiken, A. M., Nolan, A. H., Liss, S., Hogan, A., & Silkman, R. H. (1989). Evaluating managerial centers using data envelopment analysis. *Medical Care, 27*(12), 1175-1188.

Shaffer, F. (1983). DRGs: History and overview. *Nursing and Health Care, 4*(7), 388-396.

Sherman, H. D. (1984). Hospital efficiency measurement and evaluation. *Medical Care, 22,* 922-938.

Woodward, J. (1965). *Industrial organizations: Theory and practice.* New York: McGraw-Hill.

Young, D. W., & Saltman, R. B. (1983, January-February). Preventive medicine for hospital costs. *Harvard Business Review, 61,* 126-133.

Nursing Case Management to Achieve Integrated Clinical Expertise and Improved Resource Utilization

Sharon J. Coulter
Christine A. Wynd
Connie Miller
Linda J. Lewicki

Nursing case management was first introduced to this large, urban, midwestern hospital in 1988. A model of patient care management was envisioned that would provide nurses with a direct link to patient care decisions. In addition, the global health care economic climate was demanding more efficient use of resources and continuing attention to high-quality services. As the project unfolded, four phases were planned: the preliminary pilot (1990-1991), initiation (1991-1992); refinement (1992-1993), and expansion (1993-1994). A comprehensive evaluation model has incorporated attention to political, economic, and clinical impacts on issues of ownership, collegiality, and specialty expertise across departmental boundaries. Clinical and operational evaluation allows case managers to monitor patient care and progress on a daily basis, and more long-term tracking of data is used for a summative evaluation of identified patient, system, and practitioner outcomes. To date, evaluative data have revealed improvements in clinical effectiveness, as dem-

AUTHORS' NOTE: The authors wish to acknowledge the administrative staff and nursing personnel of the Cleveland Clinic Foundation, Cleveland, Ohio, for their support of this entire nursing case management project.

onstrated by quality indicator scores on seven major aspects of care, and operational efficiency, as indicated by lengths of stay (LOSs) for targeted DRGs reduced by an average of approximately 3.5 days. Total nursing costs for recommended, budgeted, and actual staffing on case-managed units have tended to be lower than on noncase-managed units.

Provision of health care in the United States is currently characterized by rapid change due to technological advances, a growing population of elderly clients, an AIDS epidemic, and larger numbers of chronically ill patients. Prospective payment strategies give insurance companies and other payers tremendous influence over patient care practices by determining standardized lengths of hospital stay (Liebman-Cohen, 1990; Safriet, 1992). Today the health care system is continuously criticized for its swollen and unwieldy bureaucracy, described as fragmented, complex, and expensive, with subsequent poor monitoring of resource utilization. In fact, the term *health care system* has been called a misnomer in that "the word 'system' connotes organization, coordination, and a considered structure, none of which accurately describes the present arrangement" (Safriet, 1992, p. 419).

For many years, the nursing practice climate has also been one of discontent and change. Nursing shortages and diminishing resources contribute to a general sense of tension, and nurses realize they are often restricted from effectively mobilizing resources for the provision of high-quality patient care. Discontent may be avoided by enhancing professional nursing practice within service settings (McClure, Poulin, Sovie, & Wandelt, 1983). Increased professional status, autonomy, control over practice, and maintenance of high-quality standards are significant factors contributing to nurse work satisfaction, retention, and productivity. Nurses want to participate in organizational systems that allow them to meet patients' needs through clinical practice decisions geared toward improving health. Nurses, who have accepted patient care responsibilities for many decades, now want to gain the authority to act in the patient's best interest.

Systemwide change is needed to improve quality care through coordination and decreased fragmentation of services. Implementation of such a change could inevitably produce the desired outcomes of improved resource utilization and lower costs. Other necessary changes include significant enhancement of nurses' images of themselves as professionals, with public acknowledgment of nurses as key partners in the provision of health care.

Work systems that foster these changes will meet the challenges of future trends. Nursing case management is a system currently receiving attention and being promoted as a framework for resolving many of these organizational issues. The purpose of this chapter is to describe a comprehensive work redesign project involving nursing case management. Theoretical rationale and operational practicalities are discussed, with an in-depth examination of program evaluation and its effect on the evolution of a nursing case management model used in one institution.

REVIEW OF THE LITERATURE

The concept of case management originally appeared in the public health arena as a means for community service coordination. For years, public health nurses managed their work by patient caseload (Grau, 1984; Weil & Karls, 1985). During the 1970s and 1980s, case management in mental health care was used as a strategy for reducing noted fragmentation of services as patients were deinstitutionalized and moved into the community. The strategy represented a "broker-of-service" model used to connect patients with necessary community resources (Chamberlain & Rapp, 1991; Crosby, 1987; Miller, 1983; Pittman, 1989).

Since the late 1980s, the popularity of case management as a concept has grown in hospital settings in which there is an explicit need for continuity, efficiency, and economy in patient care. New models for hospital case management appear frequently in the nursing literature. Common themes are patient-centered coordination of care, patient advocacy, and integration of services throughout the entire episode of illness and across all clinical settings. A general goal is to achieve excellence in clinical patient outcomes while monitoring and attempting to control the cost and utilization of needed resources. Contemporary hospital-based case management is characterized by the use of a collaborative plan (critical path) that combines the work of all health care disciplines and specifies the care, treatments, diagnostics, and interventions that should be provided within a predetermined LOS. This plan is most often assigned according to the admitting medical diagnosis, or diagnosis-related group (DRG), and includes those patients considered to be high-volume, high-cost, and high-risk (Bejciy-Spring, 1991; Bower, 1992; Pierog, 1991; Zander, 1990).

At least four nursing case management models focused on acute care delivery are defined in the literature. The primary nursing case management model originated at New England Medical Center in Boston (Stetler, 1987; Zander, 1988a, 1988b). In this model, registered nurse case managers provide direct, unit-based patient care and manage a caseload of patients across unit boundaries throughout the episodes of illness. The high cost of care, due to a limited caseload of patients per nurse ratio, and the enormous workload for nurse case managers would appear to create disadvantages.

Primm (1988) designed and described a differentiated nursing case management model combining primary nursing and total patient care while differentiating various levels of nursing practice. Associate-degree-, diploma-, and baccalaureate-degree-prepared registered nurses serve as case managers and associate case managers (Malloch, Milton, & Jobes, 1990). These nurses plan and coordinate care for a caseload of patients, whereas licensed practical nurses and nursing assistants provide direct patient care. This model presents case management as a unit-based nursing care delivery system, and there currently is a growing emphasis on models offering a broader, hospital-wide scope.

The leveled practice case management model (Loveridge, Cummings, & O'Malley, 1988; O'Malley & Cummings, 1988) allows for management of patient caseload activities by professional registered nurses. A work team of registered nurses, licensed practical nurses, and nursing assistants provides direct unit-based nursing care. This model promotes differentiated practice but further delineates the role of case manager as more managerial in nature, whereas the work team provides direct patient care.

Case management may also be approached from a business-management stance as a product line (Pierog, 1991), in which resource utilization is combined with clinical practice quality standards in a prospective, concurrent, and retrospective manner throughout the illness continuum. The bottom-line care delivery model, or service volume management approach, is described by Olivas, Del Togno-Armanasco, Erickson, and Harter (1989a, 1989b). The bottom-line care delivery model is similar to another, the product line model, because it views nursing case management as a service product that should be standardized, as closely as possible, to a resulting 100% outcome conformity. The quality process can be controlled by identifying and monitoring variables that forecast change and then adjusting when change is introduced so the service product once again conforms to the standard.

Authors promoting the bottom-line model state that inspection of patient outcomes alone is an inefficient evaluation mechanism leading to delayed improvements and missed opportunities. Instead, they propose the development of process evaluations regarding the efficient use of resource/costs (raw resources; human and material resources) for higher productivity (highest quality outcomes for discharged patients).

In this business-focused model, case management incorporates principles of payer-defined managed care with activities and concepts found in clinical practice models. However, case management is more than utilization review and the determination of "appropriate" care. Care problems are not only un-covered, identified, and defined, but also evaluated in terms of planning and problem solving for improvement of hospital productivity and enhanced patient satisfaction.

Most proponents of nursing case management identify the need for tradi-tional nurse role redefinition. Essential to the development of successful nurse case managers are high-level clinical skills combined with a working knowledge of the financial aspects of health care provision, topped off by politically astute interpersonal skills geared toward collaborative, yet assertive, management of patient care (Bower, 1992; Farquhar & Robinson, 1990; Kelly, 1992; Olivas et al., 1989a, 1989b).

It behooves nurses to develop business acumen—to value not only clinical skills but knowledge about costs and productivity, reimbursement policies, and regulations of accrediting agencies, and to learn how to apply this knowledge toward the very best patient care. All of these pieces fall into place and affect the quality of patient care as well as the operational efficiency and survival of the organization employing the nurse. Institutional administrators realize a greater return on investment in nurse case managers who are empowered with the information and authority to facilitate not only unit-based change but more extensive systemwide change toward greater organizational, operational effi-ciency.

To date, most of the literature has focused on developmental questions and theoretical dialogue regarding definitions, characteristics, and processes unique to the case management concept. Much of the evaluation work has been anecdotal versus scientifically based, with only a handful of articles reporting empirical research about nursing case management, factors influencing case management activities, and a thorough examination of outcomes. Of those studies that report research, quasi-experimental, nonequivalent-control-group, pre- and posttest designs are most frequently used. Currently, findings point to cost savings and decreased LOSs for patients who are case managed (Ethridge, 1988; Ethridge & Lamb, 1989; Liebman-Cohen, 1990).

Ethridge (1988) and Ethridge and Lamb (1989) collected and tracked data over a 2-year period and evaluated fiscal outcomes by comparing LOSs and inpatient acuity levels for case-managed versus noncase-managed patients who were hospitalized for respiratory illnesses. The researchers found not only that case management resulted in a cost savings due to decreased LOSs, but that several of the formerly high-cost DRGs became revenue generators.

Stillwaggon (1989) initiated a quasi-experimental, nonequivalent-control-group pilot study of "managed nursing care" as the intervention. The sample ($N = 100$) consisted of mothers who had delivered infants through normal spontaneous deliveries, and two groups (experimental and control; $n = 50$ per group) were compared. The researcher determined costs of nursing care through weekly time card tabulations of nursing hours multiplied by average registered nurse salaries. T tests demonstrated significant differences between the two groups $(p < .05)$. Mean nursing care hours per case were lower in the case-managed pilot group (14 hours 44 minutes versus 20 hours); therefore, mean costs of nursing care per case were also reduced for the pilot group ($160.89 versus $222.60).

Conversely, another researcher found that nursing care hours were increased for case-managed patients who had undergone cesarean sections (Liebman-Cohen, 1990; Cohen, 1991). A cost-accounting process was used to examine cost-effectiveness of patient care (Cohen, 1991), and, despite an increase in patient services and treatments, there was a reduction in the use of inpatient resources, charges, and expenditures for case-managed patients ($M = \$5,147$ per case) as compared to the control group ($M = \$6,199$ per case). Costs of direct nursing care were higher for case-managed patients ($M = \$390$ per case) than for controls ($M = \$267$ per case); however, the intensity of direct care services and increased costs did not result in higher overall expenditures for the case-managed group. In fact, due to decreased lengths of stay and increased patient turnover, a potential $1 million was saved without jeopardizing the amount of direct nursing care provided to case-managed patients.

NURSING CASE MANAGEMENT
AT THE CLEVELAND CLINIC FOUNDATION

General Description

Nursing case management was introduced to this large, urban, midwestern hospital in 1988. The global health care economic climate was creating increasing pressure for efficient utilization of resources, quality in the service provided and outcomes achieved, and satisfaction of consumers and providers. In a physician group practice environment, a model of nursing practice was envisioned that would provide nurses with a direct voice and an active partnership for managing patient care.

Following a thorough literature review, the Cleveland Clinic Foundation nursing case management program was designed. The model selected by nurse decision makers at the Cleveland Clinic Foundation combines features from the leveled practice model and the bottom-line care delivery model. The case manager is a care coordinator for caseloads of patients identified by clinical DRG case types. Emphasis was placed on standardization of all case types through critical paths, or coordinated care tracks (CCTs), and a two-tiered system was provided for coordinating and delivering care as nursing case management and managed care.

Most case managers are currently unit based, because patient case types are assigned, upon admission, to specific nursing units; however, case managers are responsible for following patients across unit boundaries throughout the entire episode of illness. This activity is particularly important due to the nature of the patients, who are often acutely ill and require movement in and out of critical care units and across clinical specialties. One variation of the model is found in the cardiac department, in which patients and case managers are assigned according to physicians and surgeons. Case managers report directly to the unit nurse manager, and a work team of registered nurses, licensed practical nurses, and nursing assistants provides direct patient care, or managed care.

Key Terms and Project Goals

Case management at the Cleveland Clinic Foundation is a nursing-directed, multidisciplinary process aimed at achieving a purposeful and controlled connection between quality and cost of care for targeted patients with high-volume, high-risk, high-cost diagnoses and/or procedures. Patients are case managed across an episode of illness as long as they remain within the purview of the medical/nursing systems of the foundation. Program goals, as enacted by case managers, include

- Establishing communication tools for collaborative care management
- Using CCTs to outline, with 80% predictability, anticipated interventions to achieve expected outcomes within specific time frames for targeted patient populations
- Targeting high-volume, high-cost, high-clinical/financial-risk patient populations
- Coordinating clinical practices across professional and geographical boundaries
- Providing frameworks for continuous quality improvement in a fiscally responsible environment
- Promoting efficient use of human and material resources through the use of CCTs
- Contributing to patient satisfaction with health care services
- Coordinating provider performance with patient outcomes

Managed care is a unit-specific, multidisciplinary process directed by unit-based staff nurses who manage the care of noncomplex patients for their assigned shifts through the use of CCTs. It is anticipated that the patient will need predictable resources while following an outlined sequence of care. When a patient varies from this predicted course of treatment, the unit case manager is called in to assist. Managed care program goals, as enacted by unit nursing personnel, include

- Assisting with the management of a patient's daily hospital progress through the use of CCTs
- Focusing the attention of all health care providers on expected patient outcomes for the specific length of hospital stay
- Promoting coordinated care by managing patients on a shift-to-shift basis across a prescriptive CCT
- Encouraging consultation between staff nurses and nurse case managers for patients experiencing variances delaying discharge or interfering with the achievement of articulated clinical outcomes, and/or variances unresponsive to interventions
- Coordinating provider performance with patient outcomes
- Contributing to patient satisfaction with health care services

Nursing Case Management Evaluation Program

A formative-summative model was selected for evaluating nursing case management (Herman, Morris, & Fitz-Gibbon, 1989). Formative evaluation represents concurrent, process-oriented monitoring of operations with opportunities for correcting problems and making improvements during program implementation. This type of evaluation is used as a source for decision making in continuous program development and improvement. It is anticipated that program design will fluctuate in response to rapid organizational change; therefore the evaluation model must account for change.

In addition to this process orientation, summative evaluation allows for the assessment and documentation of program effects, and the focus is on implementation outcomes. This component of evaluation is included to measure program successes and failures each year and to answer questions regarding program effectiveness.

Evaluation activities include specification of program goals, the program model and design, and identified outcome indicators of goal attainment (Herman et al., 1989). Goals for the evaluation of nursing case management are listed below:

- Development of case management as a collaborative process
- Development of CCTs for high-volume, high-clinical/financial-risk, high-cost patient populations
- Recruitment, hiring, and orientation of nurse case managers
- Development of an educational program related to nursing case management

- Establishment of an automated, integrated system for collecting, retrieving, and reporting outcomes data, specifically
  1. Service utilization (variances, hospital delays)
  2. Length of stay
  3. Cost data
  4. Quality indicators (clinical discharge outcomes, Medicare denials, readmissions)
  5. Human resource consumption
  6. User satisfaction (patient, nurse, physician)

The Cleveland Clinic Foundation nursing case management program has been developing and evolving for the past several years. That evolution has been chronicled in accordance with the evaluation goals.

Pilot Phase (1990-1991)

With initial objectives of enhancing quality, cost, and satisfaction outcomes, nursing case management was piloted on five inpatient nursing units from July 1990 through July 1991. Pilot study nursing units included two cardiothoracic units specializing in cardiac surgical procedures such as open heart and valve replacement surgeries, one combined medical-surgical unit focusing on otolaryngology, and two medical units representing internal medicine, gastroenterology, renal hypertension, nephrology, renal transplants, and endocrinology.

Two reports describe various aspects of the pilot study evaluation (Lewicki, 1992; Miller, 1992). Pre- and postimplementation data demonstrated that as a result of case management, clinical effectiveness, defined as quality indicator scores on seven major aspects of care, was maintained or improved, particularly in the areas of patient satisfaction, medication errors, and motion-related events. Patients were positive about receiving nursing staff support, as measured by the Nurse Support Scale (Gardner & Wheeler, 1987); however, statistically significant improvements over preimplementation data were not established.

Operational efficiency was improved because LOSs for targeted DRGs were reduced by an average of approximately 3.5 days when compared with Health Care Financing Administration (HCFA) mean LOSs. Decreased LOSs were more closely associated with surgical units, in which patient processes and outcomes followed more linear and predictable plans. Medical units had patients whose unpredictable and uncertain progress made it difficult to assign critical paths, or CCTs; yet there was a reduction in LOS for the pilot unit patients compared to all other noncase-managed patients assigned to medical units within the Cleveland Clinic Foundation (see Table 5.1).

TABLE 5.1   Effects on Length of Stay for Case-Managed Versus Noncase-Managed
            Patients (Pilot Medical Units, 1990-1991)

	Case-Managed Patients (n = 12)		Noncase-Managed Patients (n = 12)	
	Frequency	Percentage	Frequency	Percentage
Decreased length of stay	9	75	4	33
Unchanged length of stay	1	8	1	8
Increased length of stay	2	17	7	58

Total nursing costs for recommended, budgeted, and actual staffing on case-managed units tended to be lower than on noncase-managed units. This outcome was accomplished by changing unit staffing skill mix without changing total budgeted or actual staff numbers. For example, a mix of 75% registered nurses and 25% nursing assistants resulted in lower costs when compared to a unit with a skill mix of 65% registered nurses, 23% licensed practical nurses, and 12% nursing assistants.

The pilot study provided Cleveland Clinic Foundation decision makers with an introduction to nursing case management. Beginning improvements in resource utilization and clinical outcomes encouraged administrators to enlarge the number of nursing units participating in case management. In June 1991, a director for case management was appointed and began work to coordinate and refine many of the related processes vital to a program of case management. Evaluators were also brought "on board" and added a formative (process) component to the evaluation of outcome measures already in place.

Initiation Phase (1991-1992)

The current model for case management and managed care began to be implemented throughout the inpatient areas of the hospital in July 1991, as part of the Division of Nursing strategic plan. Initially, case management was monitored through updates and quarterly reports written by the chairman of the division and sent to the chief executive officer and the boards of governors and trustees. These efforts helped to garner institutional support and recognition for case management.

The chairman and the case management project director met with every medical department chairman to communicate the plan for implementing case management. All of these activities were meant to foster a collaborative process, yet the philosophy for maintaining case management within the Division of Nursing stemmed from the fact that nursing had a 24-hour-per-day patient care responsibility and nurses were the central source for 24-hour patient information. Nurses were, therefore, best equipped to coordinate multidisciplinary services.

As a beginning step for implementing nursing case management, the chairman of the Division of Nursing directed five CCTs to be developed for each nursing unit by December 1991. This goal was met and, in fact, by the end of 1992, 55% of all inpatients were managed with CCTs.

The first draft format for CCTs was piloted in April 1992. Each CCT was required to meet a standardized, single-track format for use across the Division of Nursing, with emphasis placed on correlating CCTs with the established system of nursing documentation. At the same time, it was deemed important to gear CCTs toward use by multidisciplinary professionals, patients, and their families. CCTs were, and continue to be, defined by specific patient case type and based on DRGs; they are developed in a collaborative manner with participation from all health care providers, and represent standards for measuring patient/family, system, and provider variances and delays.

The next step in the initiation phase of hospital-wide implementation was to increase the number of nurse case managers. Recruitment and hiring became an internal process as case managers were hired from available nursing personnel already employed by the Cleveland Clinic Foundation. It was deemed strategically important to maintain this new project as a budget-neutral endeavor. Though a single job description existed, there was also flexibility among nursing departments regarding qualifications for nurse case managers and their operational functions. Although centralized supervision for case management was assigned to the project director, administrative management was decentralized to clinical nursing department directors and unit nurse managers for purposes of budget preparation, hiring processes, and performance appraisals. The numbers of unit-based case managers to be hired were based on projected patient days, patient acuity, and percent occupancy. In 1992, there were 10 case managers employed by the Cardiothoracic Department, 1 case manager for Medical Nursing, and 7 hired for the Surgical Nursing Department, a total of 18 case managers within the Division of Nursing.

Case managers were required to be registered nurses with at least 2 years of direct patient care experience and prior performance appraisals denoting expert levels of practice, demonstrated self-direction, independence, and a high level of interpersonal skills. No minimal educational requirements were defined; however, a bachelor's degree in nursing was preferred. The preliminary job description was reviewed by an appointed nursing task force in May 1992 for the purpose of accurately capturing key job responsibilities. These included directing and coordinating a plan of care for a select group of patients, monitoring and evaluating that care, and managing the patients' transitions from inpatient to outpatient care and discharge.

In January 1992, a Case Management Education Advisory Group, consisting of nurse educators, case managers, nurse unit managers, clinical nurse specialists, and the project director, was appointed to assess learning needs and to plan, direct, and evaluate educational programs relevant to nursing case management. Educational needs were initially identified as defining roles and clarifying expectations for nurse case managers, ensuring channels for communication and coordination between nursing case management and managed care, marketing nursing case management to staff nurses and physicians, collecting and tracking data from CCTs, performing variance analysis, and seeing that these data were computerized. One of the major learning needs was financial information about DRGs, reimbursement systems, and billing processes. In addition, staff nurses were interested in learning about the goals and benefits of case management, differentiation of nursing case management and managed care and the impact of case management on daily bedside nursing practice.

A formalized orientation program consisting of 4-week, 3-month, and 6-month phases was also developed for newly appointed nurse case managers. The program addressed many of the identified learning needs. Two major aspects of learning for the orientation program included general principles and objectives for case management and case manager role transition. Eighty hours of nonclinical time were provided to new case managers for their orientation, and time was available for them to work with experienced case managers as preceptors.

A Nursing Case Management Automation Committee was established in March 1992 to identify data needed for clinical and evaluative aspects of case management. The committee consisted of representatives from case management, nursing research, nursing information systems, quality management, fiscal managers, and medical operations. In addition, a collaborative working relationship was promoted with the Medical Information Services Division (MISD). Therefore, case management information needs were incorporated into MISD's strategic plan.

Integration of standardized data across nursing departments continues to be an area of concern for program effectiveness. Owners of data need to be located and available data must be obtained. The next step is to design a standard method for collecting, processing, and retrieving data for analysis and evaluation.

Summative evaluation for the initiation phase examined quality clinical outcome data regarding hospital readmissions within 30 days. Noncase-managed patients at the Cleveland Clinic had a readmission rate of 15%, whereas case-managed patients at the Cleveland Clinic experienced a reduced rate of 11.7% readmissions. LOS data for the Cardiothoracic Nursing Department revealed a reduction of approximately 3,000 patient days, with a potential cost savings of over $1 million for four of the cardiac DRGs that were case managed. In addition, an institution-specific cost-comparative analysis of case-managed versus noncase-managed DRGs was performed (Konrad, Yeom, Saar, & Altus, 1992) to evaluate marginal cost effectiveness from baseline 1990 DRGs, using "a 5% inflation factor with a volume neutrality adjustment" (p. 1). Sixty-six DRGs were case managed by the end of 1991, 14,898 (49.2%) of all admissions were case managed, and 68.2% of the case-managed DRGs had a decrease in average LOS (15,956 patient days were reduced). Reductions in average direct costs per case were demonstrated in 53.8% of the case-managed DRGs, and the average direct cost per case decreased by $303.80 compared to $56.90 for noncase-managed DRGs (a savings of five times greater for case-managed DRGs). The "aggregated marginal savings" was computed to be $4.5 million for case-managed DRGs.

Initial efforts for implementing case management attempted to place the new concept in the best political and organizational light. Acceptance across disciplines was important for introducing and sustaining widespread change. One of the greatest strengths of this work redesign was that of ensuring adequate communication across disciplines with subsequent avoidance of "turf-protection" issues. Organizationally, these efforts resulted in a broad investment in case management.

Unfortunately, at the start of the project, communication within the nursing ranks was not as well emphasized, and the average staff nurse was not brought into the project until after initial implementation of case management was under way. Lack of attention to these important players limited and delayed staff nurse understanding. Nursing involvement, education, guidance, and feedback were hurriedly put into place to rectify the situation. Case management is now a large aspect of new nurse employee orientation, and the Cleveland Clinic Foundation Nursing Education Department is working with local schools of nursing to introduce case management into basic preparatory curricula.

Refinement Phase (1992-1993)

By June 1992, the case management program was implemented throughout the inpatient nursing division, with a total of 26 unit-based case managers. As the third year was entered, the complexity of collaborative relationships continued to build. A new multidisciplinary Utilization Management Team (formerly the Utilization Review Committee) was formed, and included representatives from nursing, medicine, surgery, operations, finance, and quality management. Program changes initiated by this team included moving the utilization review process from Health Data Services to the Department of Social Work, formation of a Complex Discharge Consultation Team, and a Hospital Transfer Work Group. Members of these two groups were charged with examining targeted resource-intensive patient populations and internal and external systems affecting patient discharges and transfers.

Development of a business and clinical relationship between the Cleveland Clinic Foundation and Kaiser Permanente, effective January 1993, brought additional collaborative demands for ensuring successful patient and organizational outcomes. To synchronize case managers from two very different systems, administrative nursing personnel from both organizations exchanged information and worked to achieve a seamless patient care coordination system.

In-hospital transfers across clinical departments to and from nursing units and critical care units became a challenge early in the refinement phase. Issues for coordinating case management across these boundaries were examined and a "group practice" scheme was devised for consultations among case managers caring for specific-DRG patient case types. Unit personnel first caring for the patient initiated the CCT, and that CCT was shared with "receiving" unit nursing personnel as the patient was transferred.

As of March 1993, CCTs were implemented for 240 diagnoses and procedures relating to 126 DRGs. By the end of 1993, it is expected that CCTs will be developed and implemented for DRGs comprising 80% of all patient discharges.

The recruitment and hiring of case managers has stabilized. Meetings continue to be held monthly for information sharing and for presentation of selected activities and topics contributing to individual growth and development, such as payer-based managed care, utilization review, and available alternative or allied health patient services.

Efforts continue toward full automation and integration of data required for case management. System Archive Retrieval (SAR), an on-line report-viewing system, among other systems, will allow case managers access to patient information housed on the mainframe hospital computer.

The Hospital Delay Tool (Selker, Beshansky, Pauker, & Kassirer, 1989) was piloted in 1991-1992 and formally introduced housewide in January 1993. The tool is used extensively for tracking patient/family, system, and provider variances, or delays, and inefficiencies from CCTs and patient charts. Delays are defined as unnecessary hospital days (24 or more hours). Ten categories of delays are related to test scheduling; obtaining test results; surgery; consultations; patient; provider responsibility; research, education, training; discharge planning; unavailability of appropriate level of outside care and resources; and pharmacy/medications.

Efficiency issues, or inefficiencies, are defined as occurrences when services did not actually contribute to unnecessary hospital days, but services also were not delivered within "standard" times. A codebook developed by Division of Nursing personnel assisted in the identification of eight major diagnostic categories, 45 specific procedures, and 59 consulting services (42 medical and surgical services and 17 allied health services) that could potentially contribute to patient delays and inefficiencies. In addition, physiologic variances accounted for a majority of delays and inefficiencies. Thus, the codebook also contained 19 general and 91 specific physiologic variance categories with the delay tool.

Data are collected concurrently by case managers, and compiled data reports are used to identify trends and patterns for revising CCTs as necessary, analyzing utilization management issues, "fixing" delay problem areas, and for designing practice and systemwide changes. Approximately 600 patient episodes are analyzed per month across all departments within the Division of Nursing. From January to May 1993, results demonstrate that a majority of delays are attributed to discharge planning from the patient and family perspective. Specifically, patients and families insist that patients remain in the hospital, they are undecided regarding patient disposition, or the patient has difficulty learning the information and skills needed for discharge. Another area for large delays is unavailability of outside resources for rehabilitation, skilled nursing, and intermediate care, particularly related to patients' being placed on waiting lists or evaluated by outside facilities.

Expansion Phase (1993-1994)

Various databases are being used to design system, practice, policy, and procedural changes, and unit-based quality improvement programs are established specifically to measure attainment of patient discharge criteria. Data reveal a need to move beyond the unit-based model and expand to follow the patient across the entire care continuum.

During the expansion phase, case management at the Cleveland Clinic Foundation will be extended from the inpatient hospital to the ambulatory setting. When discharged patients make their first return appointments to the outpatient clinic, an evaluation will be performed by clinic personnel to assess maintenance of discharge outcomes. Outcome failures and other problems will be directed to the case manager who was formerly assigned to the patient. The case manager will then conduct an assessment to determine reasons for failure, such as noncompliance with the medical regime, knowledge deficit, or physiologic variance. Patients who are readmitted to the hospital again become part of the case manager's caseload.

The ultimate clinical outcome measure is patient functional status, which will help to determine if case management has enabled discharged patients to regain their own level of "health" as well as the ability to function as independently as possible. A selected population of patients will be given the SF-36 Health Status Questionnaire (Ware & Sherbourne, 1992) as a measure of functional health. This 36-item self-administered questionnaire measures three health attributes: functional status, well-being, and an overall evaluation of health. Eight health concepts are also measured: physical functioning, social functioning, role limitations due to physical problems and/or emotional problems, mental health, energy/fatigue, pain, and general health perception. This tool will be administered to discharged patients during the first outpatient clinic visit.

Expansion to the ambulatory clinic represents a first attempt to define nursing case management in terms of an entire continuum of care from admission through hospitalization to discharge and outpatient follow-up. This approach offers a comprehensive evaluation of patient functional status, an attempt to maintain high quality outcomes, reduce costs, and enhance conservation of increasingly limited health care resources. Operationally, nursing case management will continue to be unit based, but conceptually, there is movement toward a patient population-based model.

Work will continue in the area of automation for linking CCTs with nursing documentation, clinical evaluative data such as the delay tool, daily fiscal/resource information, LOS data, patient acuity classification, and quality management and improvement systems. Automation will assist access to patient financial data, unit costs, and utilization review on a more timely basis to improve daily clinical practice decisions for patients across the health-illness continuum.

CONCLUSION

Bower (1992) stated that "nursing case management is not a nursing care delivery system added to existing (work) designs" (p. 17), and the experience of the Cleveland Clinic Foundation confirms this statement. Nursing case management is larger than a delivery system and requires integration and incorporation of the entire hospital organizational structure and culture. Although nursing case management may not be the only variable influencing lengths of stay and other outcome parameters, it clearly has been the driving force increasing awareness of other health care professionals concerning the need to manage resources before, during, and after inpatient hospitalization. Patients, physicians, and nurses report positive gains in continuity and consistency in patients' daily care. Early discharge planning and ongoing community referrals, key factors for increasing quality care and reducing hospital lengths of stay and readmissions, are now routinely accomplished through a multidisciplinary approach coordinated by nurse case managers.

REFERENCES

Bejciy-Spring, S. M. (1991). Nursing case management: Application to neuroscience nursing. *Journal of Neuroscience Nursing, 23*(6), 390-396.

Bower, K. A. (1992). *Case management by nurses* (American Nurses Association Publication No. NS-32, 3M, 2/92). Washington, DC: American Nurses Association.

Chamberlain, R., & Rapp, C. A. (1991). A decade of case management: A methodological review of outcome research. *Community Mental Health Journal, 27*(3), 171-188.

Cohen, E. L. (1991). Nursing case management: Does it pay? *Journal of Nursing Administration, 21*(4), 20-25.

Crosby, R. L. (1987). Community care of the chronically mentally ill. *Journal of Psychosocial Nursing, 25*(1), 33-37.

Ethridge, P. (1988). Professional nurse/case management reduces hospital costs. *Arizona Nurse, 41*(5), 1, 7, 24.

Ethridge, P., & Lamb, G. S. (1989). Professional nursing case management improves quality, access, and costs. *Nursing Management, 20*(3), 30-35.

Farquhar, S., & Robinson, J. (1990). The geometry of case management. *Michigan Nurse, 63*(5), 7-8.

Gardner, K. G., & Wheeler, E. C. (1987). Patients' perceptions of support. *Western Journal of Nursing Research, 9*(1), 115-131.

Grau, L. (1984). Case management and the nurse. *Geriatric Nurse, 5,* 372-375.

Herman, J. L., Morris, L. L., & Fitz-Gibbon, C. T. (1989). *Evaluator's handbook.* Newbury Park, CA: Sage.

Kelly, K. C. (1992). Managing care: A search for role clarity. *Journal of Nursing Administration, 22*(3), 9-10.

Konrad, D. J., Yeom, Y. K., Saar, R. A., & Altus, G. (1992). *DRG analysis 1991: A study on case managed DRGs versus noncase managed DRGs: Marginal cost savings/avoidance assessment.* Unpublished manuscript. Cleveland Clinic Foundation, Cleveland, OH.

Lewicki, L. J. (1992). *Clinical effectiveness, service satisfaction, and operational efficiency: A year-long evaluation of case management.* Unpublished manuscript, Cleveland Clinic Foundation, Division of Nursing, Cleveland, OH.

Liebman-Cohen, E. H. (1990). The effects of a nursing case management model on patient length of stay and variables related to cost of care delivery within an acute care setting (Doctoral dissertation, Columbia University Teachers College). *Dissertation Abstracts International, 51*(7), 3325B. (University Microfilms No. DA 9033878)

Loveridge, C. E., Cummings, S. H., & O'Malley, J. (1988). Developing case management in a primary nursing system. *Journal of Nursing Administration, 18*(10), 336-339.

Malloch, K. M., Milton, D. A., & Jobes, M. O. (1990). A model for differentiated nursing practice. *Journal of Nursing Administration, 20*(2), 20-26.

McClure, M. L., Poulin, M. A., Sovie, M. D., & Wandelt, M. A. (1983). *Magnet hospitals: Attrition and retention of professional nurses.* Kansas City, MO: American Nurses Association.

Miller, G. (1983). Case management: The essential service. In C. J. Sanborn (Ed.), *Case management in mental health services* (pp. 3-15). New York: Haworth.

Miller, S. A. (1992). *Case management: A pilot study and preliminary analysis.* Unpublished manuscript, Cleveland Clinic Foundation, Division of Nursing, Cleveland, OH.

Olivas, G. S., Del Togno-Armanasco, V., Erickson, J. R., & Harter, S. (1989a). Case management: A bottom-line care delivery model, Part I: The concept. *Journal of Nursing Administration, 19*(11), 16-20.

Olivas, G. S., Del Togno-Armanasco, V., Erickson, J. R., & Harter, S. (1989b). Case management: A bottom-line care delivery model, Part II: Adaptation of the model. *Journal of Nursing Administration, 19*(12), 12-17.

O'Malley, J., & Cummings, S. H. (1988). Nursing case management, Part III: Implementing case management: Operational model. *Aspen's Advisor for Nurse Executives, 3*(7), 7-8.

Pierog, L. (1991). Case management: A product line. *Nursing Administration Quarterly, 15*(2), 16-20.

Pittman, D. C. (1989). Nursing case management: Holistic care for the deinstitutionalized mentally ill. *Journal of Psychosocial Nursing 27*(11), 23-27.

Primm, P. L. (1988). Implementation of differentiated practice through differentiated case management. *Michigan Nurse, 61*(8), 33.

Safriet, B. J. (1992). Health care dollars and regulatory sense: The role of advanced practice nursing. *Yale Journal on Regulation, 9*(2), 149-220.

Selker, H. P., Beshansky, J. R., Pauker, S. G., & Kassirer, J. P. (1989). The epidemiology of delays in a teaching hospital. *Medical Care, 27*, 112-119.

Stetler, C. B. (1987). The case manager's role: A preliminary evaluation. *Definition, 2*(3), 1-4.

Stillwaggon, C. A. (1989). The impact of nurse managed care on the cost of nurse practice and nurse satisfaction. *Journal of Nursing Administration, 12*(11), 21-27.

Ware, J. E., & Sherbourne, C. D. (1992). The MOS 36-item short-form health survey (SF-36). *Medical Care, 30*, 473-483.

Weil, M., & Karls, J. M. (Eds.). (1985). *Case management in human service practice.* San Francisco: Jossey-Bass.

Zander, K. (1988a). Managed care within acute care settings: Design and implementation via nursing case management. *Health Care Supervisor, 6*(2), 27-43.

Zander, K. (1988b). Nursing case management: Strategic management of cost and quality outcomes. *Journal of Nursing Administration, 18*(5), 23-30.

Zander, K. (1990). Differentiating managed care and case management. *Definition, 5*(2), 1-3.

CHAPTER 6

Empowerment for Redesign: A Staff Nurse Perspective

Mary L. Fisher
Loraine Brown
Julie Hall
Becky Fitzgerald

This chapter describes dynamic changes staff nurse roles must undergo in a work redesign environment. The contributions of RN empowerment and shared governance to successful redesign efforts, the need for new levels of accountability for patient outcomes, and the fundamental changes in RN role under redesign are explored. Three case studies by staff nurses illustrate the creativity and potential that can be unleashed in an atmosphere of change in which staff input is sought and staff feel empowered to control their practice. These elements are essential to a successful redesign process.

Change is perhaps the most dynamic aspect of the redesign process. Some redesign efforts have focused on physical and operational changes that place services closer to the patient. To the extent that redesign focuses resources on more direct patient care activities and eliminates clerical and organizational distractions, patient-focused goals can be achieved (Borzo, 1992). But because systems are dynamic and interrelated, it stands to reason that physical reorientation also affects the human element of patient care: the nursing staff.

It is vital for a student of work redesign to understand the dynamic effect of operational redesign on the most fundamental care role, that of the registered nurse (RN). This chapter explores the evolution of RN roles within a single institution, St. Vincent Health Services in Indianapolis, Indiana, as the redesign process matured over a 4-year period. Staff nurses, through their active involvement in shared governance, have been able to assume an ever-increasing role in forging redesign plans as new units have been added to the complement of Care 2001 units, as the new model is called.

Care 2001 is the St. Vincent version of a patient-focused care model. Care 2001 looks at the patient as the center of care and is based on four principles: patient-focused care, efficiency and effectiveness, simplicity, and an environment for innovation. As staff look at issues to be resolved on the unit level, these four components are the guidelines by which decisions are made.

St. Vincent Health Services is a member of the Daughters of Charity National Health System. St. Vincent includes a 618-bed regional referral hospital, a 100-bed community hospital, a stress center, and a residential center for young adults with disabilities. Nursing followed a traditional centralized model until the beginning of the redesign process. As each nursing unit moves into the Care 2001 model, it is decentralized into a service-line model.

This chapter describes the effects on staff nurses of what Ackoff calls interactive planning (Strengthening Hospital Nursing Programs, 1992). This type of planning designs backward, from an idealized design or from guiding principles, rather than from the perspective of simply solving problems in a current system. It is a broadly participative process that is continuous. Interactive planning takes a holistic view that recognizes the need to simultaneously coordinate the process interdependently across the organization (p. 12). Many of the innovations described here are consistent with those illustrated in the Progress Report for recipients of the Pew Charitable Trusts/Robert Wood Johnson Foundation Grants to improve nursing practice (Strengthening Hospital Nursing Programs, 1992).

Through three case studies, the reader is given an insider's insight into the struggles staff nurses undergo with the elements of redesign. The role ambiguity that develops when new types of caregivers are introduced and the increased accountability for patient outcomes related to case management (referred to as *coordinated care* at this facility) are just two examples. These case studies are written by staff nurses who have grown from their experiences and are empowered to reach out for new challenges, such as writing for publication for the first time. The maturity of their insights indicates the level of professionalism that redesign demands of its nurses.

THE ICU EXPERIENCE

In the first case study, Julie Hall, an intensive care unit (ICU) clinical charge nurse (CCN), describes the introduction of shared governance to the unit. The CCN role is that of a shift leader who helps determine staffing needs while maintaining a patient care assignment of her own. As members of a pioneer unit in "Shared Decision Making," ICU nurses experienced many challenges. Trust became a central theme as staff took risks to overcome years of traditional management-staff polarization to work together in a new environment. Helping staff to build necessary skills for the challenges of both shared governance and redesign is a critical role of leaders in this model. The role of education in cross-training and team building demands a new level of institutional support for staff development.

The 32-bed ICU is staffed almost exclusively by professional nurses. Although the nurses historically functioned at a high level of clinical autonomy, they struggled in collaborating to make unit-based decisions. Sometimes traditional manager/worker relationships or day-to-day operations prevented follow-up or problem resolution. Staff felt powerless, frustrated, confused, and often angry that seemingly simple issues were not addressed and that major problems seemed too complicated for resolution.

The CCN was in the position to solve problems but often had to rely on limited staff participation. Implementation of 12-hour shifts had complicated communication. We knew there had to be a better way. The missing links were in areas such as consistency, information sharing, and ownership.

The search began for a better way to solve problems collaboratively. In 1989, the concept of shared governance was discussed at the American Association of Clinical Nurses Leadership Meeting in Boston. It was apparent that this problem-solving method would have a critical impact on the future of nursing. Managers are accountable for larger areas, assume more administrative duties, and spend less time on the unit. It makes sense to develop more professional nursing roles that allow nurses to be responsible owners of the decision-making process. Stated simply, shared governance is a formally recognized and organized system made up of professionals who accept the autonomy and responsibility of unit operations through a documented decision-making process (Porter-O'Grady, 1991).

Changing Times

The CCN began sharing her interest in shared governance with staff. They were skeptical that it could ever actually happen. Much time was spent sharing ideas and recruiting nurses who supported the process. The hospital sent the CCN to visit the Catherine McAuley Health Care Center in Ann Arbor, Michigan, to tour that facility and to explore its shared governance structure. Porter-O'Grady's work also served as a foundation for a pilot proposal that was being prepared by a task force chaired by the CCN. The proposal carefully discussed definition, goals, and objectives for the ICU and recommended a pilot model. After collaboration, the staff and manager became enthusiastic. Unit retreats were planned to finalize the proposal. Approximately 97% of the staff attended one of the four 4-hour sessions.

Wilson (1989) cites change as a major challenge in the implementation of shared governance. For us, willingness to change was gaining momentum, and trust was becoming more evident than in the past. The staff monitored attendance and shared split shifts to attend the sessions. The retreat was the first time that staff nurses had discussed ways to be autonomous, empowered, and responsible in their practice. The agenda included introduction, information, and further development and refinement of the proposed model. The more staff learned about the accountability model, the more receptive they became.

Implementation

The task force identified a framework that included five councils. The retreats were designed to provide a forum to refine goals and functions of the councils. These were opportune times for the whole unit to establish guidelines and operating regulations. Each council had a set number of seats available based on identified needs for that particular group. After nominations, the selected members chose their chair or co-chairs. Issues outlined in the regulations included length of terms, commitments to the councils, calendars, and work distribution.

Each council has specific duties. The Quality Assurance Council (QA) deals with unit-based QA issues and monitors standards of practice. The Staff Development Council is committed to facilitating unit-based educational activities. The Peer Relations Committee focuses on communication issues, recruitment, and retention. The Management Council is involved in unit operations regarding budget and resource allocation. The Executive Council collaborates with the chairs of all councils and facilitates their work.

The idea of assuming a leadership role was very intimidating to some of the staff as they became involved in the councils. A CCN sat on each of the four councils. CCNs served as nonvoting members to facilitate group dynamics and to advise in the decision-making process as needed. Council members were gently assisted to become more independent and confident informal leaders. The hospital is preparing educational programs specifically designed to develop the staff in their roles as leaders. These programs will better facilitate staff transition into shared decision making on other hospital units by providing a leadership foundation necessary for successful staff participation in unit leadership and work redesign.

Possibly the most crucial factor in the transition to shared decision making was to establish a mutual trust between staff and management. If trust had not been established early, credibility of the entire process would have been in jeopardy. The task force identified staff needs and determined their understanding of responsibility and accountability related to shared governance. The manager was very supportive and aware of changes her role would undergo with this model. Because she was participatory in her management style, she made the transition easily to an even more collaborative, facilitative role. Her supportive attitude was crucial as staff left the security of the worker/manager mentality and moved to a more responsible, empowered role.

Organizationally, change to shared decision making was supported and valued by the hospital administration. The staff needed to assume the task of redesigning unit decision making before they could fully understand the organization's trust and commitment. We had to change our level of involvement to become more actively involved in decisions before administration's traditional management style would change. In other words, we were an active influence on the administration's recognition of the contributions we could make. From this standpoint, shared governance must be a grassroots movement.

The most important aspect of the process was communication. We made no assumptions. Information was respected, and input and feedback were specific, descriptive, and timely. Team cohesion was supported, and two-way communication was reinforced. Communication became a major effort in the implementation phase and beyond.

Letting Go and Getting On

The honeymoon period started in July of 1990. We had a lot of investment in this new approach to problem solving. It was an exciting time; everyone was collaborating, meetings were being held, and there was much interaction and curiosity. Skeptics were still supporting their peers cautiously and staying involved peripherally as the informal leaders stepped forward and assumed responsibilities for initiating the change into shared governance.

Most of the seats on the councils were filled, and each council started ambitiously and rather idealistically to examine their list of goals. They were novices in the decision-making process and had little experience in group work. Once they realized the need to prioritize and distribute work, the groups were able to address issues in a more appropriate manner. At first, relatively short-term issues were addressed that could be resolved rather easily. Visible outcomes helped the groups to gain confidence and trust.

The Management Council discussed active involvement in interviewing new associates and developing an orientation program for new physicians and house staff. Council members now interview prospective associates. They are working on entrance and exit interview forms. The Management Council prepares the unit for accreditation. Staff on this council are now involved in new product evaluation and make recommendations for capital expenditures. The Peer Relations Council focused on unit communication, nurse recognition programs, and an ICU newsletter. The Executive Council, which consists of the manager, CCN, and chairpersons of the other councils, meets to review work and progress. Initially, 45% of the staff was actively participating in council work. The climate on the unit seemed to change with the success of the model. There were fewer accusations and frustrations, and there was more discussion and responsibility. The success of the first year became apparent as the chairpersons reported to the unit at the annual retreat. We were a pioneer unit to operationalize formal shared governance at our institution.

Future of Shared Governance

We continue to promote the shared governance philosophy throughout the organization. The ICU has shared their experiences with other nursing units to avoid redundant work and to facilitate the growth of shared decision making throughout the organization.

Shared governance is filtering into other non-nursing areas. Currently, Respiratory Therapy is implementing shared governance with assistance from ICU.

Because the model was instituted from the unit level up, instead of from the top down, there have been inconsistencies in its design and application from unit to unit. Developing a formal shared governance model administratively would complement the unit models so that the units could effectively network and complete the process. Such a centralized network of unit-based councils is now in the planning phase. This is especially important with the decentralization of organizational structure that is occurring with Care 2001. Several of the Care 2001 units no longer report through the Nursing Division, but through a service line manager. If we are to maintain consistent standards and customer service as decentralization develops, nurses must have an umbrella shared governance organization for communicating important issues across the institution.

A collaborative practice that involves all levels of caregivers through representative input and timely communication fosters the highest quality of care for our customers. Limited resources, competition, costs, and political regulation demand that health care organizations meet the challenge of providing autonomous practice at the bedside. After 3 years in the process, we feel successful. The current need is to remotivate and stimulate the staff so that they continue to feel productive. The annual retreat serves that purpose by communicating council work to all staff and stimulating creative approaches to clinical issues.

SETON WEST

This second case study outlines the beginning of work redesign at St. Vincent. Loraine Brown, a Professional Staff Nurse III (PSN III, the highest level of the hospital's clinical ladder for staff nurses), writes of the nurses' experiences working on the pilot redesign unit. The unit was planned from the top down, and staff were selected from volunteers in the hospital. Staff did become involved in ongoing innovation, but the basic ground rules had been set. Now, 3 years later, the unit is still evolving through the very active participation of unit staff. As former chairperson and current member of the unit's Practice Committee, Mrs. Brown especially highlights how that committee has affected the quality of patient care.

Care 2001—A New Concept of Care Delivery

In January 1990, Seton West became a reality. This unit was the first of its kind at St. Vincent. The 44-bed general surgical unit promised to be different from anything the nurses had ever experienced. The opening of Seton West, the first Care 2001 unit, began St. Vincent's commitment to redesign the current delivery system and to focus on changing our paradigms in many ways.

This new change soon became a way of life for the staff of Seton West. The structure of the unit looked different from any other in the hospital. Instead of having the typical central nursing station, the unit was divided into six substations. Patient-focused care became possible by bringing services closer to the patient. On Seton West, the patient rooms are stocked with patient medications and supplies needed for daily patient care and treatments. The staff have been cross-trained to perform certain activities at the bedside, such as EKGs, phlebotomy, respiratory care, and order entry. Because staff can perform more patient services, they spend more time with patients than before (Brider, 1992).

The unit also houses a laboratory where cross-trained staff perform frequently ordered labs and an X-ray room where routine X rays are performed when a licensed radiologic technologist (RT) is available. The patients are admitted directly to Seton instead of through the central admitting area. Chart coding for billing purposes also is decentralized to the unit.

The Team Concept

Another difference that Seton West encountered was that the RNs and LPNs were asked to invite a new role into the patient care delivery component, that of the technician (tech). The techs came from a variety of backgrounds; some had previously worked as phlebotomists, EKG techs, RTs, or X-ray techs. They were trained to give patient care and perform other cross-trained skills. The tech role provided a huge challenge for nurses who had never worked with anyone other than licensed personnel, but it also enabled nurses to value the wealth of knowledge that could be shared through these relationships. Many of the nurses now depend on the information that can be obtained from the experiences of these techs. An EKG tech was a godsend when performing the first real EKG, and it is wonderful to have a phlebotomist who can always access that patient who is a really hard stick.

The staff of Seton West grew as a team. The team concept is the driving force behind Seton's success. But although it sounds wonderful on paper, it is not always peaches and cream in reality. The staff have been involved in many role clarification and team-building workshops to facilitate the process of the team concept. The nurses have had to learn new ways to lead their teams more effectively.

Shared Governance

The staff of Seton West has gone through many changes, perhaps the largest dealing with the unfamiliar shift to a shared governance model versus the old "I do what I'm told" role. Instead of seeing management as the control of the unit, the staff has become empowered to make decisions and solve problems. The role of the manager becomes a teaching, coaching, and mentoring role. The staff role becomes a professional role that focuses on problem solving, participating in the decision-making process, working in collaboration with others, and becoming involved in peer evaluation and hiring new staff.

The catalyst of Seton's shared governance model is Seton Council and committees that branch off the council. These committees are similar to those described in the first case study, with the addition of the Lab Core Committee. The Lab Core Committee maintains the unit lab, making sure that the Lab Core team members are up to date on their check-offs and knowledge level of the lab procedures. The accomplishment of the Practice Committee will be highlighted to illustrate how much growth the nurses have experienced.

Practice Committee Contribution

The Seton Practice Committee has brought about many changes for the unit. The first milestone that this committee has accomplished is developing standing orders for the surgical and urological patient populations. The standing orders have helped the nurses develop autonomy and have increased their decision-making skills. To implement these protocols, physician involvement was crucial. Representatives from this committee began a collaborative effort with physicians by attending their section meetings and asking for feedback. The relationships between the nurses and physicians have improved not only through discussing standing order issues but through experiencing the entire Care 2001 concept as well. The physicians play a valuable role in supporting positive changes on this unit as well as molding future units into the Care 2001 model.

The Practice Committee is currently working on promoting and implementing the coordinated care (CC) program on Seton West. CC at St. Vincent is a collaborative process between patient and health care team to maintain or improve patient outcomes while managing resources effectively. CC uses the tool of a care map/critical pathway in order to achieve the following goals:

1. Enhance patient and family participation with care by sharing information from critical pathways and providing appropriate education.
2. Facilitate optimal patient outcomes within appropriate lengths of stay.
3. Promote professional development and satisfaction of the health care team.
4. Direct contributions of the health care team toward achieving optimal patient outcomes.
5. Promote appropriate utilization of resources.

The process of making CC successful and meaningful to the RN is an on-going process. With major changes occurring in our health care system today, it remains a challenge to focus our efforts on patient education and to prepare patients for self-care at home. Seton is utilizing critical pathways for patients who have undergone the following surgeries: laparoscopic cholecystectomy/appendectomy, transurethral resection of the prostate/bladder tumor, nasal septal reconstruction, and tonsillectomy and adenoidectomy. The presence of these pathways have empowered the RNs to play a larger role in determining how patients will progress during their hospital stay as well as after they are released.

A formal research study has been developed as a result of the implementation of CC on Seton and the Orthopedic Unit. "A Comprehensive Outcome Evaluation of the Coordinated Care Program" will be evaluating many aspects of CC, such as cost, length of stay, the patient's functional ability and perception of nursing care, associate satisfaction, and the time it takes to give report on a patient who is on a critical pathway. The results of the study will validate the effectiveness of CC.

Tackling Documentation Dilemmas

Traditional operations utilize 29% of nursing staff time in documentation (Borzo, 1992). Charting must be streamlined along with other redesign efforts to reduce time spent on documentation and increase time staff can have available for direct patient care. Staff nurses from Seton and other nursing units have developed a new form that concentrates on "problem, implementation, and evaluation" focused charting (PIE). Input from staff and physicians was sought before beginning the pilot, and revisions are still in progress. The new format allows the reader to look quickly at a coded assessment versus a hand-written narrative assessment. Only the patient's active problems are written in the narrative section of the chart form, followed by implementation and evaluation. This method of charting has increased the accountability of the RNs, encouraging them to look at the patient's problems more thoroughly than in the previous system.

Conclusion

The staff on Seton continue to grow and face new challenges daily as we move toward nursing in the future. The concept of Care 2001 is here to stay. We now must concentrate on delivering quality patient care through a shared decision-making model that fosters continuing innovations.

5 WEST

The final case study, written by Becky Fitzgerald, shows how staff have evolved to become central to the planning of changes in redesign today.

Because the 5 West staff had already matured in their shared decision-making model, they were poised to take a very active role in defining their unit, both with designing physical changes and with role development. Miss Fitzgerald's position, practice facilitator, is a new role designed by the staff on her floor with the leadership of their unit manager. This position is much more of a clinical resource than the previous position of clinical charge nurse.

It is critical to note that staff from other Care 2001 units (to date there are seven) helped in planning this unit. The sense that it is important to learn from past models and to further evolve the concept is classic to the redesign process. The story about this third-generation redesign unit is important from the aspect of shared governance and interdisciplinary involvement.

Beginnings of Change

Acceptance of change by staff can be very difficult to achieve. The attitude of management and the involvement of staff in the planning and education for change play a large part in the acceptance of that change. When unit-level management promote change in a positive light, and when staff are well educated and involved in planning for change, the result can be the vested interest of staff in the successful achievement of change on a nursing unit.

We first heard of patient-focused care (Care 2001) when the hospital planned the trial Seton unit in 1989. Our unit's conversion began in the fall of 1992, with the unit opening in early January 1993. This time span allowed the staff to learn more about patient-focused care and helped them assimilate the change.

This is not to say that everyone embraced the concept of Care 2001 with open arms. A few resisted it, many were skeptical, and others had a wait-and-see attitude. A few associates even decided to leave the unit rather than accept the coming change to patient-focused care.

Changes were already occurring on our unit along with changes toward patient-focused care occurring in other parts of the hospital. We had begun a shared governance model in early 1990 and had active committees in place by the time we began training in 1992 for Care 2001. Having shared governance up and running was a help in the staff s acceptance of the change toward patient-focused care.

One drawback our unit faced was that we were changing not only our patient care delivery system but also our patient population. We were originally a medical unit and would be converting to a neurovascular focus.

Although we had nurses with excellent clinical skills, most felt uncomfortable with the prospect of caring for this new patient population. An added stressor was the fact that our 38-bed unit would also contain a 9-bed acute neurovascular unit. The type of care on this unit within a unit would be between progressive and intensive care. We would be doing everything except ventilator support and arterial lines. This would add to the training that our staff needed in addition to the normal cross-training provided in preparation for Care 2001.

Pretraining

The unit's Education Committee stepped in and became very proactive in working with the Care 2001 education staff that would provide training for patient-focused care. These two groups began working together about 9 months before we began formal training. An outline for our training was the result of this joint effort.

Because the patient population was changing, we needed to establish an adequate neurological background. The unit's Education Committee enlisted many of the hospital's neurologists to assist with staff educational needs. The physicians presented a series of lectures on various diagnoses that would be admitted to the new unit. These lectures were taped and became mandatory viewing for all licensed staff. The tapes also will be used in the future by new associates to help ensure a consistent and solid basis for neurological patient care.

The Education Committee, in conjunction with the Quality Improvement Committee, started a subcommittee to begin work on critical pathways. It was felt that using the care maps would help ensure consistent quality care for the new patient population. The ideas that came out of this subcommittee grew and expanded into more and more projects, with the end result being the formation of a new and separate committee, Coordinated Care.

The Coordinated Care Committee did extensive research about critical pathways during this time. A few units throughout the hospital were using them in a limited manner. We were much more ambitious, with the goal to have critical paths ready to use for the seven most frequently admitted diagnosis-related groups (DRGs) by the time the unit opened in January 1993.

A new neurological flow sheet was developed that coordinated with one used by the ICU. This would help provide continuity of care and help the staff to recognize subtle changes in a patient's neuro status. New changes were occurring with the nursing care flow sheets throughout the hospital. The committee also became involved in this project, contributing input about the charting needs of our unit.

Because all this documentation was new and was developed by the unit's associates, the Care 2001 Education staff was unable to provide the training for this area. Therefore, members of the Coordinated Care Committee provided extensive training in the use of the critical pathways, the neuro profile flow sheet, and the new charting forms during cross-training. Now, after opening the unit, the committee still is involved with auditing the various chart forms to assess for any changes or further education that may be needed.

In August 1992, a task force was formed to look at the entire issue of patient-focused care at St. Vincent. By this time three units had been through training and unit renovation and were operating under the Care 2001 model. There still was resistance to the concept by some physicians, nursing staff, and various ancillary departments. The task force was developed to help resolve the conflicts, to reiterate the reasons for the change to patient-focused care, and to develop a prototype model for the successful change over to Care 2001 by the rest of the hospital.

The task force was made up of representatives from administration, ancillary departments, nursing staff from Care 2001 units, and physicians. Subgroups were formed, with associates from our unit serving as members or chairs of the committees. The needs of our new patient population were evaluated, and decisions were made on how to best meet those needs.

We convened a multidisciplinary group whose mission was to focus on patient care. The first goal was to develop a multidisciplinary assessment form so that each patient's need for referrals could be identified at admission. Further work of this group has resulted in the unit's adoption of twice-weekly multidisciplinary conferences. The ultimate goal as this practice matures is to focus on measurable benefits for patients and their families.

The Peer Review Committee also was busy during the period prior to our entering training. Part of patient-focused care was the incorporation of bedside technicians, cross-trained to perform patient care as well as technical tasks. This committee became involved in interviewing applicants for these positions and had input into the eventual hiring of the new staff. The goal was to have these new staff members hired, through their bedside training, and assimilated into the larger group of the unit prior to entering the cross-training phase. Other units had found that delays in hiring their techs resulted in a "us versus them" attitude that delayed formation of a cohesive work group and interfered with the team building that was needed.

One benefit for the existing staff in being able to interview and hire these new associates was seeing the enthusiasm of these people who wanted to work on the unit. They voiced positive attitudes about our unit and Care 2001 that resulted in a feeling of pride and a more positive view of patient-focused care. Another outcome of the staff s involvement in hiring new associates was their responsibility for those new associates. It was harder for staff to complain about someone if problems arose, but they easily could take credit for a great staff when things went well.

As the time for training approached, most of the staff were anxious to begin. They had been extensively involved in the change process, so their opinions had been incorporated into the final plan for the unit. The staff now had a vested interest in the outcome of this change process and wanted to see it succeed.

Training Begins

In October 1992, the training planned for so long began. Training itself was a challenge for several reasons. It had been years since many of the staff had been in a classroom setting. The idea of listening to lectures and taking tests was a stressor for many people. Now everyone was thrown together 5 days a week, 8 hours a day. This was a change in everyone's schedule and resulted in an adjustment in the staff's lifestyles as well as those of their families. The staff missed patient contact and were anxious to get back to the bedside by the time training was over.

One thing we had wanted to work on during training was role clarification. While everyone was in training, we wanted to define the roles of RN, LPN, and tech, differentiating between what each could and could not do as defined by state law. This ended up being a very difficult task, with tempers flaring and feelings hurt. During training, 10 hours were spent in small groups and all together trying to come to an agreement about what each role meant and how roles worked separately and together. We still struggle with these questions at times, perhaps because the cross-training allows all levels to do similar tasks. It is harder to articulate the more professional aspects of the RN role. People tend to define themselves by the tasks they do and not by the mental processes necessary for professional judgment.

Another problem anticipated after the unit opened was achieving credibility with the physicians. The goal was to increase communication between unit staff and all the physicians. One complaint physicians had about Care 2001 was that they could never find the nurse who was taking care of their patient. (Happily, this was because the nurses were now with the patients and not in a nurses' station.) We worked very hard before and during training to develop a communication plan to increase interaction. The RNs began carrying cellular phones so they could respond directly to physician calls. Other communication solutions were designed by the Core Group. This committee included one physician from each admitting group (family practice, internal medicine, neurology, neurosurgery, and vascular), RNs from the unit, and an RN from ICU. The purpose of the group was to provide communication between staff and physicians, to make decisions, and to act as problem solvers.

A result of this attempt to improve relationships between physicians and nurses has been an improvement in collaborative practice. There have been many compliments from the physicians who practice on Five West. The interaction helps provide better care for our patients and helps to increase nurses' satisfaction with their jobs.

End of the Beginning

Our unit has undergone tremendous changes in the past few years, and the positive effects on the unit and the associates are a direct result of the effort that was invested. We were fortunate to have a unit manager who guided and encouraged staff to grow professionally. We were allowed to empower ourselves by developing a shared governance model. This surely helped prepare staff for facing the challenges of converting to a patient-focused neurovascular unit.

The effort put out by each person on the unit was not equal, and one cannot expect it to be. Because of personal commitments and each nurse's experience, some could be more involved than others. Those who were ready and wanted to grow professionally were the ones who worked the hardest and therefore gained the most personal satisfaction from the experience.

Even now that the unit is up and running, the change process is not complete. Staff still grapple with some of the problems encountered before and during the unit conversion. Even though most of the physicians have been pleased with the changes, some have not. Staff continue to try and meet their needs because they are our customers in addition to the patients. We also continue to work with the ancillary departments, discussing new issues and refining procedures that were found ineffective when put into operation. Ongoing role clarification is an identified need as efforts are made to help each individual strive toward his or her potential.

The staff have experienced a rare opportunity to participate in creating a new nursing unit. Their ideas were valued; their suggestions were used. The staff are invested in this new unit, and they are proud of the result.

CONCLUSION

This chapter has presented three examples of the impact of work redesign on RN roles. The level of involvement required of professionals in this more decentralized model of decision making requires the institution to invest in the human elements of redesign. Not only do technical functions change, but the very nature of professional practice is affected. O'Malley and Llorente (1990) recommend that redesign efforts maximize the use of professional nurses at a level more consistent with their role potential.

Nurses must be assisted to more fully develop professional leadership skills. Many nurses who are accustomed to functioning more independently in a primary nursing model need to learn delegation skills for the first time. The concept of the team as more than individuals working independently requires work. A consistent team that takes time to work through superficial issues to develop a higher level of functioning is a real benefit to be gained from the redesign process. There are tremendous efficiencies to be obtained from such synergistic relationships. A team that can truly work together can accomplish more than loosely bound individuals. They view the work as a team effort and may not even accept individual assignments. Each worker in this type of team solves problems as they arise rather than passing them up the line. Customers receive more direct and prompt benefits from people operating under this patient-focused philosophy.

An atmosphere that supports innovation and risk taking is essential to successful redesign. These characteristics and strong central administrative support were cited as essential components to effective planning in a study of the planning processes used by participants in the Strengthening Hospital Nursing Program discussed earlier (Taft, Jones, & Minch, 1992). Staff can become actively involved in making the system better when they feel secure enough to risk. This was illustrated very well by the contrasts among the three case studies. As staff became more empowered within the shared decision-making environment, the institution benefited by a broader input in the planning process. The nursing staff are the clinical experts. They are the people closest to the customer. They are very much aware of what supports practice and what inhibits clinical effectiveness. What institutions must learn to do is listen to the real experts. Then the health care system may be able to face the challenges of a system that is out of control, and patient outcomes may become the central focus of those efforts.

REFERENCES

Borzo, G. (1992). Patient-focused hospitals begin reporting good results. *Health Care Strategic Management, 10*(8), 16-23.

Brider, P. (1992). The move to patient-focused care. *American Journal of Nursing, 92*(9), 26-33.

O'Malley, J., & Llorente, B. (1990). Back to the future: Redesigning the work place. *Nursing Management, 21*(10), 46-48.

Porter-O'Grady, T. (1991). Shared governance for nursing: Creating the new organization. *AORN Journal, 53*(2), 458-466.

Taft, S. H., Jones, P. K., & Minch, E. L. (1992). Strengthening hospital nursing, part 2: Characteristics of effecting planning processes. *Journal of Nursing Administration, 22*(6), 36-46.

Strengthening Hospital Nursing Programs. (1992). A program to improve patient care, gaining momentum: A progress report. St. Petersburg, FL: Author.

Wilson, C. (1989). Shared governance: The challenge of change in the early phases of implementation. *Nursing Administration Quarterly, 13*(4), 29-33.

CHAPTER 7

A Three-Dimensional Model for Planning and Documenting Care

Susan L. Peterson

Care plans have been an unattested requirement for over 50 years. In actual nursing practice, care plans often are not properly documented, are not utilized in the delivery of care, and as studies have shown, they have no significant effect on patient outcomes. Nurses at Columbia Hospital, Milwaukee, Wisconsin, utilized continuous quality improvement methods to study this problem. They found that nurses did not utilize care plans in the delivery of care because the content of the document was already part of the nurses' knowledge base. Nurses typically learn to write care plans as an educational tool rather than as a communication tool. A three-dimensional conceptual model of planning was created that is the foundation for designing alternative documentation methods. An implementation project is discussed that has resulted in the elimination of care plans, the development of a planning flow sheet supported by clinical guidelines to standardize patient care, a reduction in nursing documentation time, and increased nursing satisfaction.

It is time for nurses to revolutionize structures, processes, and systems in nursing and health care. Sovie (1989) defined the term *revolutionize* to mean radical change as opposed to evolutional or more gradual change. To accomplish this, individual nurses must be empowered to create new and better ways of providing nursing care. Nothing should escape scrutiny, examination, and evaluation. "Nurse administrators and managers need to legitimize the slaughtering of sacred cows and facilitate the radical changes as well as support the continuous evolutionary changes that are required to maximize nurses' time for quality care" (Sovie, 1989, p. 79). Nurses must discard what does not work or produce desired results, and many suggest that one of the first rituals that should be examined is the care plan (Davis, 1993; Frank, 1988; Otterman, 1991; Palmer, 1990; Sovie, 1989).

Nurses have attempted to find the solution to the care plan challenge for over 50 years. Originally implemented as a teaching aid in the 1930s (Ackerly, 1939; Blunt, 1937), the care plan evolved into a frustrating professional practice component as the escalating requirements for documentation competed for the time nurses had to care for patients (de la Cuesta, 1983; Shea, 1986). It has become an administrative nightmare to balance the need for regulatory compliance with the need to reduce nursing time involved in paperwork, while still integrating various documentation puzzle pieces to form a clear picture of the patient's care (Daniel & Fulmer, 1992; Hegland, 1992; Worthy & Siegrist-Mueller, 1992). Over time, the care plan has changed: Nursing diagnosis has been added, it has become a permanent part of the medical record, and it has been computerized. Nurse administrators have repeatedly tried to change nurses' attitudes about care plans by appealing to professionalism or enforcing care plans as a standard through quality assurance monitoring and performance evaluation.

What has not changed, however, is that after nurses graduate and enter the workforce, they may find that skillful development of care plans using the model learned in the educational setting is not useful or practical (Gwozdz & Del Togno-Armanasco, 1992). As they become more experienced, they do not view traditional care plans as useful because the written information is already a part of their knowledge base. In the end, they perceive the care plan as an onerous task to be accomplished within the already limited time they have for documentation. More often than not, they either do not complete it or do it solely to meet administrative requirements. This chapter documents the efforts of one hospital to meet the challenge of planning and documenting care efficiently and effectively through the development and implementation of a three-dimensional model for planning care.

HISTORY OF THE PROBLEM

The Nursing Department at Columbia Hospital, a 394-bed facility located in Milwaukee, Wisconsin, tried most of the improvement strategies mentioned and was still unsuccessful in consistently meeting care plan documentation requirements or satisfying nurses' requests for streamlined documentation methods. A nursing theoretical model had been adopted, a book containing standard care plans had been published, and the entire process for documenting care plans had been computerized. Managers received automated reports identifying which patients did not have an active or current care plan and counseled staff nurses who were not in compliance. In 1986, a documentation survey was done that included questions focused on the care plan. The survey was returned by 158 nurses, or 56% of the staff. Nurses were asked to rank chart forms in three categories on a scale from 1 to 7. The responses indicated that of 15 different documentation forms, the care plan was considered of least value in reflecting care given and the needs of patients. It was also identified as the most difficult form to use (Columbia Hospital, 1986). Many improvements were made to the overall documentation system between 1987 and 1989, but the care plan continued to be criticized by staff and managers alike.

The computer became the next logical focus for improvement. In 1989, another survey was conducted examining the automated care plan system. Nurses self-reported spending an average of 19.3 minutes per shift initiating or updating care plans for their assigned caseload (Columbia Hospital, 1989). Most comments indicated that the computer was difficult to use, so the hospital attempted to work with the computer vendor to design system changes. Each proposed solution, however, was either cost-prohibitive or not technologically feasible.

By this time, the care plan problem had been studied by myriad groups and individuals, and no solution could be identified. The complexity of the problem was overwhelming. Symptoms included software that was not user-friendly, fragmentation in documentation, redundant communication methods, lack of a common understanding of use of the nursing process, and variation in patient care practices used from unit to unit. Most of all, there was intense nursing frustration with spending valuable time writing a care plan that was not valued because it was considered unnecessary in the delivery of patient care.

A Shift in the Diagnostic Journey

In 1991, the hospital became influenced by the philosophy of continuous quality improvement (CQI). Once more, a task force was reassembled, and, by the methods of continuous quality improvement, the root cause of the care plan problem was recognized and identified. Issues were brainstormed, the flow of the process was studied, and a cause-and-effect analysis technique was used to create a breakthrough in thinking. It became evident that all previous problem resolution efforts had been aimed at symptoms rather than the root cause of the dilemma. The new problem statement was simply phrased, "The care plan is not used." The group knew, however, that competent patient care was being delivered even though the care plan was not used because of acceptable quality assurance, risk management, and patient satisfaction feedback. It was clear that the reason the care plan was not used was that it did not contain useful information.

Although it was not available to the group at the time, the task force recognized what was later documented in a study by Hildman and Ferguson (1991). Nurses needed a communication tool for planning and delivering care, not the complex process document used in the educational setting.

With this breakthrough in thinking, the group decided that developing care plans was a non-value-added nursing activity that should cease. A project mission statement was created that read, "Design an alternative method of documenting the planning of patient care." The goal was to find a documentation solution that would serve as a communication tool, would stand the test of actual use by nurses in their practice, and would meet regulatory requirements. Although group momentum had increased, the first of several hurdles was yet to be crossed. Their proposal to stop doing traditional care plans was based on assumptions that needed to be validated. The necessary support was found in the literature.

Studies on Care Plans and Patient Outcomes

In reviewing the literature, it was noted that there is much information on how to write better care plans but little exploration on whether they have any impact on patient outcomes. Ferguson, Hildman, and Nichols (1987) studied three types of care-planning systems and their impact on patient outcomes. They discovered that there was essentially no effect on length of stay, number of readmissions, rate of nosocomial infections, number of incident reports, number of medication or treatment errors, number of controlled drugs administered, and acuity level on discharge; nor was length of shift report affected for any one of the care-planning systems. In addition, there was no significant impact on patient satisfaction. The conclusions of this study were relevant to our project for two reasons. First, the researchers suggested that the process of identifying nursing diagnoses and interventions is a cognitive process. It is based on the nurse's education and experience and does not require a written form to be available to deliver quality care. Second, planning care is only one step of the nursing process, and it is the sum of all of the steps of this process that influences patient outcomes. To separate the planning phase from the entire nursing process in not logical.

A study by Aidroos (1991) contained a blind evaluation of 158 psychiatric patients with and without care plans over a 5-month period. In this study, the quality of care was judged to be higher where a care plan either did not exist or was not followed. It was postulated that this was due to greater independent practitioner judgment being put to use in the care of patients. Another study compared computer-supported and manually generated care plans developed for patients with AIDS (Holzemer & Henry, 1992). In addition to finding no difference in patient outcomes between the two systems, there was a discovery made in the study that nearly one third of the sample populations did not even have a documented care plan. Therefore, it may be assumed that this subgroup also experienced no difference in outcomes.

Changes in Standards in Care Planning

At about the same time that these studies were appearing in the literature, the Joint Commission on Accreditation of Healthcare Organizations (JCAHO, 1991) was rewriting nursing standards. These newly revised standards did not specifically require a care plan. Instead, documentation in the clinical record needed to include identification of patient needs, interventions, care provided, and patient response or outcomes. This freedom from needing to mechanistically write a care plan, combined with our chief nursing executive's openness to not being tied to the current computer system, empowered a group of nurses to think about planning in a new way. They created a conceptual model of planning that in turn drives new methods for documenting the planning of care.

THE REMEDIAL JOURNEY

The original task force was joined by an optimal mix of staff nurses and nursing leadership members to form the Design Group. The diagnostic work and research findings were reviewed, the problem statement was supported, and commitment to the mission was attained. Using methods of continuous quality improvement, an accelerated process improvement technique, and the concepts of creativity and change, the group designed the solution and implementation plan within three highly productive workshop days during the third quarter of 1992.

They first adopted the assumption that the planning phase of the nursing process is cognitive work, not clerical work, and that because of this, care plans do not have an impact on patient outcomes. They determined that the perception that writing care plans detracts from patient care stems from the fact that writing down what you plan to do for a patient is redundant with what you already know in your mind you will do for a patient. The primary reason for documenting the plan should be to communicate to other caregivers what is not known about a specific patient's care needs rather than what they already know. The group realized that planning care should more closely resemble a prescription of interventions for a specific patient whose care needs are outside of a typical standard of care.

The study phase of the care plan problem had lasted nearly 3 years, so a solution was long overdue. Three workshop days were planned to accelerate the typical process improvement methods of continuous quality improvement. In the first session, creative brainstorming resulted in 68 alternative methods of communicating a patient's plan of care. These were grouped into 10 categories by a sorting technique called the affinity process. Decision-making criteria developed by the Nursing Practice Council were assigned priority through each member of the Design Group's interviewing of 10 staff nurses as part of their prework for the workshop. Additional criteria thought to be missing were added. Ultimately, 11 criteria were agreed upon, some of which were considered critical in the selection process. By using two critical criteria, (a) "complies with regulatory standards" and (b) "affordable in fiscal year 1993," the list of options was pared down to 42. These remaining options were posted to a matrix tool called a critical grid and ranked on how well they met all 11 criteria. The resulting scores were analyzed, and the top 7 options were retained.

On the second workshop day, anxiety surfaced and became a barrier to further decision making. A question was raised that the group had difficulty answering: "What type of planning do we need to document?" In a discussion about planning, the nurses felt that there were different degrees or types of planning activities conducted throughout the course of patient care. It was acknowledged that planning occurs from admission to discharge and, with shorter hospitalizations, begins at preadmission and may extend to postdischarge. Some planning is as simple as timing the administration of an analgesic prior to a painful procedure; other planning is as complex as arranging teaching for a newly diagnosed diabetic patient who is blind. Planning may occur in a fleeting moment as a nurse assesses a wound and mentally leaps through the planning phase of the nursing process so quickly that interventions have already been determined. It may also consist of a routine prescription for care that seldom varies, which sometimes is referred to as a standard care plan or critical pathway. To make a quality decision, the group needed to better define planning; a conceptual model was needed. This was the driving force behind the development of the Three-Dimensional Model of Planning Care.

Three-Dimensional Model of Planning Care

Little and Carnevali (1976) describe planning as an "active decision-making process in which consideration of the relationships between goals, actions and consequences (outcomes) precedes taking action" (p. 8). Planning is the pre-

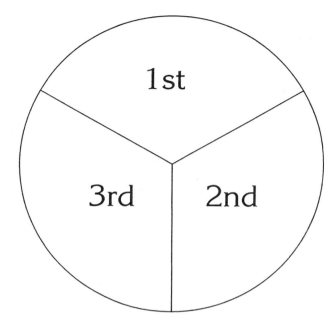

1st Dimension: Clinical Guidelines
2nd Dimension: Nursing Orders communicated to oneself in thought only
3rd Dimension: Nursing Orders that need to be carried out over time or need to be
                 communicated to others

Figure 7.1. Three-Dimensional Model of Planning Care
SOURCE: Model created by Care Plan Design Group at Columbia Hospital 1992.

scriptive process that may be communicated as an order to oneself in thought
only, or to others. The nursing order or prescription for care has the intent of
individualizing care for a particular client at a particular time. The nursing
order is explicitly differentiated from other closely related plans used by the
nurse, specifically, a standard care plan. The standard care plan deals with the
commonalities. Nursing orders should address what is different, not what is
the same.

The three-dimensional model of planning care (see Figure 7.1) carries
through on that theme while incorporating the findings of the research described earlier. The model inherently assigns value to the nurse as a knowledgeable professional by recognizing that care of patients is more than a series of
procedures and activities. Planning is not defined as a phase with a starting and
ending point, but rather as an ongoing cognitive aspect of patient care that
nurses frequently have not articulated well to each other, let alone to the patient.

The lack of recognition of this analytical process causes us to think of planning as simply a list of things to do that can be written down and checked off when completed. What needs to be affirmed is the nurse's skillful ability to assimilate scientific knowledge, experiential knowledge, and a concurrent assessment of the patient's condition immediately into a plan of action.

The three modes of planning depicted in the model are (a) clinical guidelines, (b) nursing orders communicated to oneself in thought only, and (c) nursing orders to be communicated to other caregivers. The intent and method of documenting each of these dimensions of planning are different. The nurse may draw upon one or all three dimensions at the same time in a critical thinking process in determining what to do next for a patient.

Clinical guidelines are standard plans for the management of nursing care associated with certain medical and/or nursing diagnoses or clinical conditions. The term *guidelines* was chosen to remain consistent with the American Nurses Association's (1991) language regarding nursing standards and with the Agency for Health Care Policy and Research (AHCPR) Clinical Practical Guidelines. Guidelines describe the techniques and observations that constitute the commonalities of care for a group of clients. Guidelines communicate to staff the patient care expectations that standardize nursing practice and ensure continuity of care for patients. For the novice nurse, they may also serve as an educational tool or resource support during orientation to the professional role. Guidelines may be documented and stored as a collection in a manual, a computer database, or some other form. The specific guideline applicable to a patient needs to be referenced but not physically contained in the medical record. This is similar to the systems in place for documenting and retaining nursing policies and procedures. They, too, are part of a plan of patient care but are only referenced in the chart.

Nursing orders are prescriptions for individual client care needs that supplement or modify the standard of care (Carnevali, 1983). Nursing orders are frequently communicated to oneself in thought only and then are carried out by the nurse. It is typical for a nurse to modify the plan of care or prioritize interventions differently, based on the patient's assessment as the nurse is implementing the plan. For example, the nurse may decide to do one patient's teaching before ambulating him because he will be too exhausted after the activity to learn well. These nursing orders are referred to as the second dimension of the model. When the nurse documents such assessments and interventions, this presumes that preplanning has occurred as a cognitive process that does not require a written plan of care. Documentation of what was done and how well patient needs were met is sufficient for this realm of planning.

Other nursing orders need to be carried out over a period of time or may need to be communicated to other caregivers. An example could be the specific pain control regime that works for a patient prior to a physical therapy treatment. These nursing orders make up the third dimension of planning. They need to be recorded within some type of communication tool so that they are incorporated into ongoing care of the patient.

The Model Drives the Documentation Solution

The three-dimensional model of planning care was the result of a major shift in thinking. The model gave the Design Group a uniform framework to draw from in completing their decision making. Each member now had a clear, common understanding of planning. The group quickly agreed that existing nursing standards of care would fit with the first dimension of the model but would need to be revised substantially. Current flow sheets and other chart forms could continue to be used to document care described in the second dimension of the model. It was the third dimension, nursing orders that needed to be communicated to others, that would require a documentation vehicle not yet in place.

Before the conclusion of the second workshop day, a final decision was reached. A tool called matrix prioritization was implemented. Each of the seven options was compared to the other six on how closely it met the criteria. The list of criteria was considered too long to keep this process manageable, so a multivoting technique helped set priorities and weight the top five criteria. An effective documentation method would be characterized as (a) simple to use, (b) easily altered/updated, (c) easily implemented, (d) compatible housewide to nurses, and (e) used by nurses. The format that most closely met the criteria was a one-page planning flow sheet.

During the third and final workshop day, the group drafted the planning flow sheet (see Figure 7.2). They also outlined an implementation plan after spending time reviewing change theory. The flow sheet design turned out to be very simple. A box is provided for recording the title only of the clinical guideline(s) selected for the patient. The remainder of the form consists of columns for documenting other patient needs, nursing interventions, and expected outcomes. One question that still had to be dealt with was whether it was acceptable for a planning flow sheet to contain only the clinical guidelines in use for a patient without subsequent documentation to prove individualization of patient care needs. There was agreement that this was both appropriate and compliant with external regulations. Individualization of care occurs on admission when the nurse determines which clinical guideline(s) apply to a specific patient, and throughout the continuum of care. It is possible that a patient

PLANNING FLOWSHEET

PRIMARY NURSE	ASSOCIATE NURSE	UNIT
PRIMARY NURSE	ASSOCIATE NURSE	UNIT

Date / Initials	Guidelines in use	Date Guideline no longer in use	Comments

PAGE ________

Date / Initials	Focus / Problem	Interventions	Expected Outcome	Date Focus / Problem Resolved

Signatures and Initials ________________________________

____

Figure 7.2 Planning Flow Sheet, Columbia Hospital, 1993

will progress as expected and that the interventions outlined in the clinical guideline will be sufficient to guide caregivers. If alterations in interventions need to be communicated to other caregivers or carried out over time, documentation of this individualized care on the planning flow sheet is appropriate. In addition, continuous individualization of the plan of care occurs on a moment-to-moment basis in the form of nursing orders, communicated either to oneself or to others, as nurses consider the patient's condition and determine new or modified interventions.

IMPLEMENTATION OF THE MODEL

The implementation plan for the project outlined by the Design Group contained three milestones for success: (a) collect feedback and refine the draft of the planning flow sheet, (b) create organizational readiness for the change through extensive communication, and (c) develop the clinical guidelines. It was this last milestone that would take a significant amount of time and expertise of others in the organization, but was also a key in improving and standardizing nursing practice. The project was guided by the Design Group, but the implementation activities were carried out by committees and councils already in existence within the shared governance model that had been in place in the Nursing Department. The Nursing Documentation Committee refined the draft of the planning flow sheet and wrote procedures for its use in a pilot project. All councils received a presentation on the model and the flow sheet. During the mid-1992 visit of the JCAHO, the nurse surveyor was consulted on the proposed way of documenting. The feedback was positive and encouraging. The Nursing Standards Committee revised its membership and purpose statement and outlined the overall scheme for developing the clinical guidelines. Early on, there existed agreement that like patient populations, cared for in geographically different units, should receive consistent care. This previously had not been the case. For this to be accomplished, some guidelines would need to be developed by groups of units. This took a longer time to accomplish, but the result has been rewarding. Nurses working within the same unit began discussing appropriateness of care; nurses from different units started working collaboratively to identify the best way to care for patients in order to provide consistent, standards-based care. This has also promoted greater alignment between ambulatory and inpatient nursing practice so that, across a continuum of care, patients may have a congruent experience in their health care.

Each nursing unit was given a template of what a clinical guideline should look like and was asked to determine how long it would take to complete the majority of guidelines applicable to the patient populations that they cared for.

TABLE 7.1 Reported Documentation Time

	Baseline Data (19 Days) November 1992	Pilot Experience (21 Days) August 1993
RN self-reported time in minutes required to initiate, update, or evaluate the plan of care per shift per assignment	19.3	5.6
Percentage of patient records containing a documented plan of care within required postadmission time frame	50%	71%
Percentage of patient records containing a documented plan of care at discharge	65%	90%
Average number of pages generated per day to support the system	240	32

The goal was to have all units using the new planning flow sheet by the end of 1993. Two units first selected to pilot the new methods were the Birthing Center (postpartum and nursery) and the Medical-Surgical Oncology Unit in June and July of 1993.

Evaluation of the Pilot Project

Several evaluation methods were used 2 months after the pilot began. These included a staff nurse survey, closed chart reviews, concurrent chart reviews, and an assessment of other areas affected by the change (e.g., the medical records function). The findings of the evaluation were analyzed along with baseline data collected prior to the pilot project. The data collection methods were not strictly comparable; however, there were some noteworthy results.

The self-reported average time spent in documenting planning dropped from 19.3 minutes per nurse per shift to 5.6 (see Table 7.1). The time savings multiplied by the average number of nurses scheduled to work each day equates to 30.6 hours of care per day gained for direct care of patients.

In concurrent chart reviews, a planning flow sheet was completed with the required postadmission time frame on 71% of the charts screened. This was a 21% improvement from prepilot experience. One of the two pilot units did achieve 98% in this area. The other unit did not have a smooth implementation and was found to have more difficulty in achieving this goal. It is assumed that with a better implementation on subsequent units, a higher success factor will be achieved. A planning flow sheet existed on 90% of discharged patients in the pilot. Compared to baseline data, this was a 25% improvement. In addition, closed chart reviews demonstrated a desirable link between the plan of care and other documentation. When a planning flow sheet existed in the record, the progress toward expected outcomes was documented and could be tracked in 95% of charts.

In a survey evaluating the overall satisfaction with the new planning flow sheet, 79% of nurses reported a score of 3 or 4 when using a 4-point Likert scale, with 4 indicating a high degree of satisfaction. Three more of the decision-making criteria related to ease of use and implementation were evaluated. Using the same scale, 89% of staff nurses found the planning flow sheet easy to update or alter, 95% found it simple to use, and 95% stated that it was easily implemented.

Other operational improvements were also noted. The medical records department experienced a reduction in the waiting period for plan of care documentation to reach the chart of a discharged patient. The former computer care plan summary took 2 days to reach the record, whereas the planning flow sheet was available immediately. This may contribute to improving chart turnaround time for billing purposes.

The volume of paper for daily working copies of care plan, management reports, and final chart copies using the automated system was an average of 240 pages per day. The pilot experience suggests that this will drop to a single chart form per admission in most cases, or approximately 32 pages total per day. This will reduce paper purchase and recycling expenses as well as the volume in the stored record.

Based on the pilot project data, housewide implementation was recommended with a few minor modifications. The inservice for nurses will contain more emphasis on documenting nursing orders on the planning flow sheet that occasionally were found on a kardex in random observations. The staff nurse questionnaire will have some statements reworded for clarity before being used again. Strategies will be identified to ensure that the flow sheet is consistently retained in the record at discharge rather than periodically discarded as was suspected during the pilot. In addition, the current system is manual due to the limitations of the existing hospital computer system, so the goal for the future would be to automate it again.

CONCLUSION

Improving quality and value are consistent messages facing health care and nursing organizations. Typically, value is sought by reducing surplus costs and scaling back on services. Unfortunately, this can result in the reduction of quality as well. Another approach is to examine practices that do not add value or do not achieve what they are thought to achieve. For half a century, nursing care plans have been considered a valuable exercise that would serve to guide quality of nursing care delivery. In reality, they may only be a helpful educational tool for the student or novice who is without the knowledge base and set of professional experiences that the practicing nurse uses to care for patients. Care plans, as they have evolved, have not been a valuable communication tool for the experienced nurse. Instead, they are mindless, repetitive documentation activities that have little impact on the quality of care patients experience.

Many have sought the solution to this dilemma but have only applied a band-aid to the problem. The three-dimensional model of planning care offers a new way for nurses to think about planning. It helps to clear confusion and to value the cognitive work often taken for granted. Documentation solutions that fit a particular nursing organization can be identified using the model as a framework. For example, critical pathways might be used instead of the clinical guidelines selected in this pilot project. The model would remain constant, but the methods of implementing it would vary. With time and more study, it is anticipated that the three-dimensional model of planning care and its application to nursing care delivery will demonstrate that breaking old mind-sets can produce radical change in the way nurses practice. This, in turn, can reduce wasted nursing resources and increase recognition of professional competence.

REFERENCES

Ackerly, L. (1939). Steps in planning nursing care. *American Journal of Nursing, 39,* 192-195.

Aidroos, N. (1991). Use and effectiveness of psychiatric nursing care plans. *Journal of Advanced Nursing, 16,* 177-181.

American Nurses Association (1991). *Standards for clinical nursing practice.* Kansas City, MO: Author.

Blunt, K. H. (1937). Nursing plans: An aid in clinical teaching. *American Journal of Nursing, 37,* 528-529.

Carnevali, D. L. (1983). *Nursing care planning: Diagnosis and management* (3rd ed.). Philadelphia: J. B. Lippincott.

Columbia Hospital. (1986). *Documentation survey.* Milwaukee, WI: Nursing Administration.

Columbia Hospital. (1989). *Care plan study.* Milwaukee, WI: Nursing Administration.

Daniel, D., & Fulmer, R. (1992). The documentation dilemma: An integrated solution. *Home Healthcare Nurse, 10*(6), 41-44.

Davis, D. (1993). Toward successful compliance with JCAHO standard NC. 1. *Nursing Management, 24*(4), 50-51.

de la Cuesta, C. (1983). The nursing process: From development to implementation. *Journal of Advanced Nursing, 8,* 365-371.

Ferguson, G. H., Hildman, T., & Nichols, B. (1987). The effect of nursing care planning systems on patient outcomes. *Journal of Nursing Administration, 17*(9), 30-36.

Frank, K. M. (1988). Tromping troublesome traditions. *Nursing Economics, 6*(6), 282.

Gwozdz, D. T., & Del Togno-Armanasco, V. (1992). Streamlining patient care documentation. *Journal of Nursing Administration, 22*(5), 35-39.

Hegland, A. (1992). Making the pieces fit: Consistency is key in care planning and charting. *Contemporary Longterm Care, 15*(6), 74-77.

Hildman, T. B., & Ferguson, G. H. (1991). Registered nurses' attitudes toward the nursing process and written/printed nursing care plans. *Journal of Nursing Administration, 21*(10), 20, 33, 45.

Holzemer, W. L., & Henry, S. B. (1992). Computer-supported vs. manually-generated nursing care plans: A comparison of patient problems, nursing interventions, and AIDS patient outcomes. *Computers in Nursing, 10*(1), 19-24.

Joint Commission on Accreditation of Healthcare Organizations (JCAHO). (1991). *Accreditation manual for hospitals.* Oakbrook Terrace, IL: Author.

Little, D. E., & Carnevali, D. L. (1976). Nursing care planning (2nd ed.). Philadelphia: J. B. Lippincott.

Otterman, S. (1991). How to make care plans work for you. *RN, 54*(8), 19-21.

Palmer, P. N. (1990). An obituary for the nursing care plan. *AORN Journal, 52,* 499-500.

Shea, H. L. (1986). A conceptual framework to study the use of nursing care plans. *International Journal of Nursing Studies, 23*(2), 147-157.

Sovie, M. D. (1989). Clinical nursing practices and patient outcomes: Evaluation, evolution, and revolution (legitimizing radical change to maximize nurses' time for quality care). *Nursing Economics, 7*(2), 79-85.

Worthy, M. K., & Siegrist-Mueller, L. (1992). Integrating a "plan of care" into documentation systems. *Nursing Management, 23*(10), 68-72.

CHAPTER 8

Planning for Patient Care Teams: A Shifting Health Care Paradigm

Virginia Del Togno-Armanasco
Sue Harter
Judith Jones

In response to the rapidly changing health care paradigm, Tucson Medical Center (TMC) has begun to restructure its patient care process. Building on a collaborative case management program that coordinates care with all disciplines and support services, TMC has started a redesign process that places the patient in the center of all care delivery activities. Direct care delivery support has been implemented through the rebundling of care delivery activities into two reconfigured roles that decrease fragmentation of care and inefficiencies of services. These are a patient service associate (PSA) to provide hospitality services and a direct patient care partnership composed of an RN and a nursing assistant with expanded skills. Specific tasks and skills redeployed and the didactic and experiential learning process required to implement these positions are described. Financial information and consumer satisfaction outcomes are presented along with anticipated continued redesign changes.

The modern hospital was essentially designed between 1900 and 1920.
—Peter Drucker (1992)

The past decade has recorded the beginnings of a major shift in the health care paradigm. The patient care delivery model is transforming from one in which the system and organization are designed around the needs of care providers to a framework that places the patient at the center of all care delivery decisions and activities. Lee and Clarke (1992) reported that the service structure of today's hospital is operationally complex and fragmented. They further noted that its structure is dysfunctional in that it is organized according to operational specialization and not according to the way patients' needs can be met. This has resulted in a high level of transaction processing and other nonvalue-added costs, with only 19% of all activities directly related to patient care (Lee & Clarke, 1992).

Murphy (1992) wrote that "hospital workers spend as an average 31% of their time overcoming roadblocks to services and cross-functional coopera-tion" (p. 9). Examples he cited include clerical and communication activities, role confusion and fragmentation, inappropriate assignment of work respon-sibilities, and structural territoriality. Thus Kohles and Donaho (1992) stated that the solutions for health care inefficiencies lie in restructuring the process.

Many facilities today are responding to the demand to improve continuity of care and reduce fragmentation. Examples of hospitals in the forefront of this activity include University of Utah, Salt Lake City, Utah; Beth Israel Hospital, Boston, Massachusetts; St. Luke's Hospitals, Fargo, North Dakota; Lee Memo-rial Hospital, Fort Myers, Florida; Sentra Health System, Norfolk, Virginia; Lakeland Regional Medical Center, Lakeland, Florida; John C. Lincoln, Phoe-nix, Arizona; and Robert Wood Johnson University Hospital, New Brunswick, New Jersey.

PROCESS OF PATIENT CARE REDESIGN

In 1991, Tucson Medical Center (TMC) embarked on this process of patient care redesign and began reassessing its current patient care delivery model to resolve these challenges. At the time, a multidisciplinary collaborative nursing case management system was in use on some units and in the implementation phase on others. Therefore, the new patient care delivery model was envisioned as one that would support the case management efforts and incorporate the economic and practical realities of our health care community, culture, and environment. These realities included a 70% and growing capitated payer mix, one thousand-plus medical staff members, a seasonal census, a nursing staff composed of greater than 60% associate degree nurses, and a rising patient

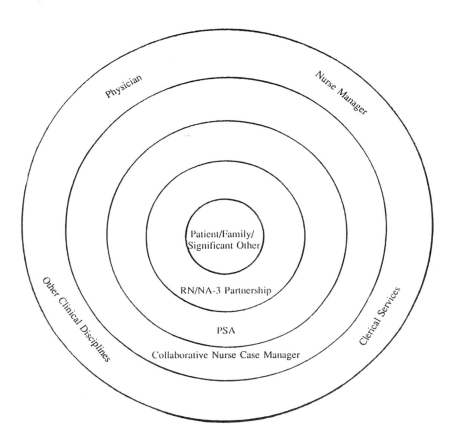

Figure 8.1. Model of Restructured Patient Care Delivery System

acuity. In addition, TMC serves a multicultural patient population including, a significant number of Mexican nationals whose English proficiency is limited.

Figure 8.1 represents our vision of the restructured patient care delivery system that could achieve these goals. It places patients at the center of all care delivery activities, with their well-being and outcomes of care receiving first priority. Surrounding the patient/significant-other dyad are the daily care providers: the RN/NA-III partnership (responsible for the daily clinical care) and the patient service associate (PSA) (responsible for meeting the patient's nonclinical needs). Coordinating care for the episode of illness is another professional nurse, the collaborative case manager. The case manager works with all clinical disciplines and support services facilitating efficient and effective individualized care delivery.

This redesign, placing the patient at the core of health care delivery, is a significant departure from the traditional patient care delivery system, in which processes are often developed for the convenience of health care providers, not the recipients of care. Employing this design as our vision, our challenge became how to implement this restructured care delivery.

The PSA Role

Our first step in the change process was to rethink and redefine the present care delivery roles. A task force made up of key nursing managers was convened to assess the current nursing care delivery roles. The task force membership included professional nurses from several patient care delivery units. Literature on nurse assistive personnel was reviewed (Alexander, 1992; Bernd, 1992; Bernd, Kern, & Wharton, 1993; Farris & O'Day, 1993; Feutz-Harter, 1988; Johnson & Miller, 1992; Kohles & Donaho, 1992; Lathrop, 1993; Leander, 1992; Lee & Clarke, 1992; Murphy, 1992; National Council of State Boards of Nursing, Inc., 1987; Ritter & Tonges, 1991; Stephens, Jones, & Watson, 1993; Tonges, 1989a, 1989b; Urmy, Dubree, & Spinella, 1993; Yarbrough, Tornabeni, & Scott, 1993; Zimmerman, Crosier, & Taylor, 1993). Taskforce representatives also visited Riverside Hospital in Toledo, Ohio, to learn about a new category of worker that combined some dietary, housekeeping, and nonclinical nursing care responsibilities.

On the basis of the information obtained, the task force next evaluated whether such an assistance worker could be instituted at TMC. We began by identifying tasks currently provided by professional nurses that could be ac-complished equally well by a less skilled worker. These tasks were classified as basic amenities or hospitality services. Examples included preparing patients for meals, delivering and picking up food service trays, and other nonclinical tasks such as taking patients to the car at discharge, making unoccupied beds, distributing drinking water and pitchers, providing snacks, answering patient call lights, and delivering flowers and mail.

Bundling these tasks into one job responsibility was perceived as especially beneficial to our redesign of patient care in that historical data from our customer satisfaction questionnaire had documented good outcomes in all but three areas: timely answering of patient call lights, keeping the bathrooms clean, and ensuring that the hot food was hot when received by the patient. We theorized that we would achieve significant improvement, as documented in our patient satisfaciton questionnaire, in these factors with the creation of this new role. Improving patient satisfaction in these areas also facilitated admin-istrative support. The outcome of our efforts was a recommendation that TMC develop a multifaceted worker to meet these basic hospitality needs.

Recognizing that such a person would perform multidisciplinary tasks, some of which were not currently within the scope of nursing responsibilities, we expanded the task force's membership to include representatives of both environmental and food services. In a collaborative process, we reached consensus as to the patient care support role, the title (patient service associate), the job responsibilities, a training program, and units that would serve as our alpha sites. We also negotiated reallocation of full-time equivalents (FTEs) from all three departments to maintain a budget-neutral position. The budget decisions were based upon a matrix listing each task, which discipline currently provided the service, time required per unit of service, and frequency of service delivery. Time required for each task was then measured and tabulated to determine the total time being spent by each discipline on each task per patient per day. Using the average daily census, we converted these totals to hours per nursing unit that each discipline would contribute to this new role. Tables 8.1 and 8.2 provide examples of these data.

Table 8.3 lists the role responsibilities of this new worker (PSA), and Table 8.4 lists the major points of their 10-day training program. Each discipline assumed responsibility for teaching the educational component with which it had the greatest involvement and expertise. This assisted in developing a rapport with and commitment to the new category of worker.

RN-NA-III Partnership

With the achievement of unanimity on a role to address the service needs of our patient and family customers, the task force next worked to identify a system to assist the professional nurse in daily care delivery. We believed there were opportunities to be gained in caring for more acutely ill hospitalized patients using a partnership concept. Again we scrutinized the literature and collaborated with friends and colleagues. As a result, the task force recommended the implementation of a patient care delivery partnership composed of a professional nurse and a nursing assistant with expanded skills. The choice of the additional skills was based on evaluation of what tasks were appropriate to delegate to the advanced nursing assistant partner (NA-III) according to the Rules and Regulations of the Nurse Practice Act of Arizona (R4-19-402). Table 8.5 lists the basic skill expectations for all NA-IIIs regardless of unit assignment.

To meet the unique needs of some patient care units, additional unit-specific special skill lists for individual units were developed. Table 8.6 identifies examples of additional special skills for a variety of specific nursing areas.

Because nursing education has focused on the delivery of primary and total patient care for the past 20 years, we recognized that there was a large cohort of nurses needing team-building and dyad-leading skills. Inasmuch as there

(text continued on page 105)

TABLE 8.1 Examples of Tasks Identified as Appropriate for Patient Service Associate

Service	Percentage of Patients Served per Day			Frequency per Patient per Day	Minutes per Service	Minutes/Patient per Day		
	Alpha Unit A	Alpha Unit B	Alpha Unit C			Alpha Unit A	Alpha Unit B	Alpha Unit C
FS Inpatient: menu completion/pick-up	90	90	65	1	.8	.7	.7	.5
ES Seven-step cleaning: semiprivate	70	37	80	1	14.0	9.8	5.2	11.2
N Soiled linen removal	100	100	100	1	1.5	1.5	1.5	1.5
FS Meal follow-up: patient satisfaction	100	100	100	3	.3	.8	.8	.8
N Patient requests: paper/water/mail/etc.	10	40	43	1	1.0	.1	.4	.4
ES Bed making: discharges	18	23	43	1	15.0	2.7	3.5	6.5
FS Nourishment delivery	22	15	100	2	1.0	.4	.3	2.0
N Move patient/discharge	18	23	35	1	25.0	4.5	5.8	8.8

NOTE: N = Nursing; FS = Food Service; ES = Environmental Services.

TABLE 8.2 Reallocation of Hours for Patient Service Associate Role

Service	Alpha Unit A	Alpha Unit B	Alpha Unit C
Hours/patient day	1.04	.86	1.44
Minutes/patient/day by service unit			
Nursing	42.78	32.18	60.74
Food service	1.91	1.77	3.27
Environmental Services	15.80	16.36	19.85
Hours/patient/day by service unit			
Nursing	.71	.54	1.01
Food Service	.03	.03	.05
Environmental Services	.26	.27	.33
Average daily census	32	37	35
Total daily hours reassigned to PSA per unit			
Nursing	18.61	11.80	21.16
Food Service	.03	.65	1.14
Environmental Services	6.87	6.00	6.91

TABLE 8.3 Role Responsibilities of the Patient Service Associate

Category of Assignment	Examples of Tasks
Patient orientation	Using the phone, television, radio, heat and air conditioning systems; calling for assistance; adjusting the bed and bedside table; storing clothing and securing valuables; requesting books, newspapers, magazines
Meal services	Delivering breakfast, lunch and dinner; feeding patients; cleaning and removing trays; providing additional food support (ketchup, utensils, salt, ice); recording caloric intake; menu completion and pick-up
Room cleaning	Making the bed; cleaning and adjusting counters, tabletops, window coverings; sweeping and washing floors; cleaning bathroom lavatory, sink, shower; emptying garbage cans; refreshing rooms
Patient transport	Exercising patients; delivering to therapy, medical services; walking to library, cafeteria, visiting rooms; admitting and discharging
Linen service	Removing soiled linens; changing sheets, pillows, mattress and pillow covers, blankets; securing additional linens; maintaining linen stock in patient's room
Nursing Assistance	Cleaning and replacing bedpans; answering call lights; talking with patient; assisting with turning, lifting; removing medical equipment upon discharge; assisting with weighing, bathing, oral hygiene, infant feeding, diaper changing
Patient assistance	Filling requests for newspaper, water, mail; watering plants; reading books, letters, memos; writing letters, notes; assisting visitors
Beverage service	Delivering and serving water, coffee, juice, ice; removing beverage service items
Translation	Speaking and reading foreign languages; assisting patients and visitors with language barriers

TABLE 8.4   Ten-Day Educational Program for the Patient Service Associate

Program Days	Content Focus	Content Topics
Day 1	Introduction of program	Identify program expectations, paradigms, and perceptions. Team development.
Day 2 through Day 4	Food service training	Detailing food service operational policies and procedures, modified diets and diet therapy, good health and nutrition, supplementation, and food handling and sanitation.
Day 5 and Day 6	Patient care orientation	Training for nonclinical nursing duties, infection control, risk management, patient transportation, hospital safety, death and dying issues, and aging awareness. CPR certification.
Day 7 and Day 8	Environmental service	Detailing seven-step cleaning procedure, chemicals and equipment, body substance precautions, and infections and hazardous wastes. Starting "hands-on" job training.
Day 9 and Day 10	Hands-on training and review	Application of skills learned in each area and interaction with staff on unit.

would be role changes for both members of the partnership, staff-developed classes were developed for each participant group. For the professional nurse partner we provided a day of didactic and experiential learning on the topics of collaboration, coordination, team building, and conflict resolution. Table 8.7 lists the class content for the professional nurse partner.

To assist the NA-III to obtain the necessary technical skills, a 2-day class including both didactic and experiential learning was also provided. Tables 8.8 and 8.9 list the educational schedules for the NA-III partner.

To promote teamwork, the members of the partnership selected each other, and only staff who wanted to practice this patient care delivery model were included in our initial classes. Support and commitment of the nursing leadership group were demonstrated by each alpha unit's nurse manager teaching one component of the class schedule for both groups.

Furthermore, the professional nurse partner of each team participated in the classroom teaching of the prospective NA-IIIs. They further participated by supervising skill proficiency of their NA-III partner in the skill laboratory and on the unit. We recommended this supervision should continue for a minimum of three times, or longer if the RN partner evaluated the need to continue past this minimum. These actions were taken to facilitate the trust relationship needed in the partnership.

TABLE 8.5 Basic Role Responsibilities of Nurse Assistant III (NA-III)

Category of Assignment	Examples of Tasks
General nurse assistant competencies (NA-I & NA-II)	
Catheterization of urinary bladder, male/female	Foley, straight, and minicatheterization; manual irrigation; discontinuance of Foley; continuous bladder irrigation, including changing bag and measuring and recording fluid intake and output
Wound management	Wet to dry dressings; packing of wound; clean and unsterile dressing change; and sterile dressing change
Specimen collection	Urine cultures catheterization; gastric pH; wounds; nasopharyngeal cultures; drainage system culture, including catheters, Jackson Pratt, and hemovacs
Gastrostomy feedings	Checking for placement of tube, manual irrigations, adding to present feeding, and intermittent feedings
Nasogastric feeding tube	Checking for placement, manual irrigations, and discontinuance
Tube feeding—intermittent (bolus) and continuous	Checking for residuals, completing irrigations, changing tubing, adding to present tube feedings, and intermittent feedings
Blood glucose monitoring	Use of Accu-chek equipment
Oral, nasopharyngeal suctioning	Oral and nasopharyngeal suctioning
IV	Monitoring drip rate and discontinuing IV
Monitoring pulses	Apical, apical-radial, pedal, carotid
Documentation of care provided	Recording care on appropriate medical record form
Intake and output	Recording intake and output of patient
Antiembolic stockings	Measurement and maintenance of hosiery
Sequential compression device	Application of and discontinuance
Observing and reporting status of ostomy site	Applying colostomy appliances, irrigating established colostomy (not new), and monitoring patient performance

TABLE 8.6 Special Unit Role Responsibilities of Nurse Assistant III (NA-III)

Area of Service	Examples of Tasks
Transitional Nursery	
Gather newborn data	Vital signs, chemstrips, and hematocrit
Perform daily care activities	Initial bath, initial feeding, and "First Foto" picture
Report signs and symptoms of neonatal emergencies	Apnea, dusky spells, respiratory distress, hypoglycemia, and hypothermia
Demonstrate safe use of equipment	All equipment used in unit
Facilitate parental/ infant interaction	Parental contact and breast feedings
Mother/Baby Unit	
Assist with baby care	Provide parent information packet; assist with breast feeding and formula feeding; teach safety, diapering, bathing, clothing, use of bulb syringe, circumcision and cord care; assist with obtaining car seat at discharge
Provide special care for infant	Perform infant bulb suctioning, positioning, and infant formula feeds; assist with circumcision, breast pump use, PKUs; and provide subsequent care for the infant receiving phototherapy
Provide special care for mother	Blood pressures, lochial cultures; auscultation of fetal heart tone; reinforce teaching parents to take their own pulse
Postcoronary Care and Coronary Care Unit	
C-clamp stasis	
Monitor pulses	Apical, radial, apical-radial, femoral, pedal, popliteal, and carotid
Swan-Ganz	Set up transducer flushes
Endotracheal tube/tracheostomy suctioning	Retape endotracheal tube and irrigate endotracheal tube as indicated
Specimen collection	Venipuncture

OUTCOMES

Our early results from the PSA program documented an annual savings on the alpha units of $35,600 and an increase of 8.4 FTEs. Of that amount, $2,700 was from a reduction in professional nurse hours, as many nonclinical tasks

TABLE 8.7 Class Content for Professional Partner

Content Area	Examples of Topics Covered
Program overview	Roles and purpose of the program, how the NA-III is to function when the RN partner is not present, and role of RN back-up partner
Communication	Managing change, conflict resolution, effective communication techniques, supportive behavior, and positive feedback
Management	Decision making, delegation, teamwork, and evaluation
Teaching	Adult education techniques, learning styles assessment, and review of the skills to be taught to the NA-III
Group discussion	Issues raised during the workshop and evaluation

TABLE 8.8 Class Content for NA-III Partner—Day 1

Content Area—Day 1	Examples of Topics Covered
Program Overview	Roles and rules of the program, how the NA-III is to function when the RN partner is not present, role of RN back-up partner, ways to support the program, and effective communication skills
Aseptic technique	Identify the importance of aseptic technique; emonstrate the techniques of aseptic technique
Documentation	Discuss the NA-III role in documentation, review the legal nature of documentation, and review the method of flowchart documentation
Obtaining cultures	Review the technique of obtaining cultures and processing culture specimen from urinary catheters; nasogastric and gastrostomy tubes; nasopharynx; and wounds and wound drainage system
Sequential compression device	Demonstrate the application, removal and maintenance of the sequential compression device; discuss the NA-III role in reinforcing patient teaching.
Accu-chek	Identify the technique of finger stick and glucose monitoring using the Accu-chek system
Skills laboratory	Skills laboratory for cultures, Accu-chek and sequential compression device
Pulses, doppler, and antiembolic stockings	Demonstrate the techniques of pulse assessment (apical, carotid, pedal, and use of doppler); demonstrate the technique of measurement, application, and patient teaching for use of antiembolic stockings
IV observation and discontinuance	Review the NA-III role in IV therapy and the technique of IV catheter removal; discuss complications of IV catheter removal and actions to take if complications occur; review calculating IV fluids for intake and output
Skills laboratory	IV and pulses

TABLE 8.9 Class Content for NA-III Partner—Day 2

Content Area—Day 2	Examples of Topics Covered
Review and questions	Content of Day 1
Wound and ostomy care	Demonstrate unsterile and sterile dressing changes, wet to dry dressings, and packing and removal of packing; demonstrate application and removal of ostomy appliances and colostomy irrigation; discuss complications that may be associated with dressing changes and actions to take if complications occur; discuss NA-III role in patient teaching
Urinary catheterization	Demonstrate catheterization of the female and male patient, use of the minicatheter equipment, and manual bladder irrigation; discuss role in continuous bladder irrigation, complications and difficulties that may occur when catheterizing the patient and action to take if difficulties occur
Nasogastric tubes, gastrostomy tubes, tube feedings	Discuss the technique of assessing tube placement, administering a tube feeding (continuous and intermittent, and nasogastric tube removal; demonstrate manual irrigation of feeding tubes; discuss complications that may occur with tube care and actions to take if complications occur
Suctioning	Demonstrate the technique of oral and pharyngeal suctioning; discuss care of the patient being suctioned and complications of suctioning and actions to take
Skills laboratory	Catheterization, nasogastric tubes, feeding tubes, and suctioning
Documentation	Review documentation of NA-III tasks
Written examination	Assess knowledge
Summary, questions, and evaluation	Clarify issues and questions regarding the new role

were redeployed to lower skilled workers. This allowed the professional nurse to spend more time on the nursing process and coordinating patient care. Immediately, patient satisfaction was documented by letters and comments to staff and administration expressing appreciation for having a person available to meet their basic needs. An example of a comment we received concerning the PSA program is the following:

I am a hospital-trained RN, and once in a great while you meet an individual completely dedicated to his profession. Besides the wonderful attention I receive from [name of PSA], he was outstanding in his attention to a little Mexican lady, Juanita, who seemed completely disoriented. He spoke Spanish to her, fed her patiently, and I must say her response to [name of PSA] was amazing. She looked him straight in the eye and carried on a conversation. (Patient)

Staff members also appreciated the support provided by the PSA. An example of such a comment is the following:

I have been pleasantly surprised by the helpfulness and availability of PSAs throughout the floors. Whether it is assistance finding a step-stool to help a patient back to bed or an extra hand in a questionable transfer, the PSA has been there when needed. I think they deserve the "Most Valuable Player of the Year" award. Thanks for starting this program, and I heartily endorse continuing it. (Physical Therapist)

Testimonials regarding the benefits of the NA-III program included the following:

This is a *wonderful* program. The NA-III has improved his clinical skills and communication with the entire staff. The partners involved in the program work extremely well together. These particular people are all clinically competent, easy going, and willing to try new things. I feel this has been an extremely positive program. I hope it continues. (RN not included in a RN/NA-III partnership dyad)

I really like the feeling of teamwork. Working together with the same people all the time allows for team building. I also find that even though we routinely have five to six patients each, I have more time to actually talk to my patients and yet I usually leave work on time, which is not usual. (RN partner included in a RN/NA-III partnership dyad)

I feel like I'm really helping the nurses when they are so busy. Also all the nurses have been very helpful especially my preceptor. Also I feel like I'm really part of the team now. They all give me respect which makes me want to do all I can for them. (NA-III partner in a RN/NA-III partnership dyad)

FUTURE EXPECTATIONS

Now we are ready to extend our work redesign. A multidisciplinary task force has been convened to examine how to continue our quest to restructure additional services and processes around the patient. It is anticipated that this may involve using less skilled workers to deliver certain job responsibilities and that new systems may need to be developed to meet these needs. Our vision includes expanding both the PSA and RN/NA-III partnerships to include more multiskilled tasks. For the PSA role we anticipate expansion to include some basic clinical tasks such as vital signs and clinical assistive activities.

For the RN/NA-III partnerships we anticipate expanding their responsibilities to include other technical skills such as phlebotomy; basic respiratory, physical, and occupational therapy; EKGs, and perhaps basic laboratory analysis. These actions are compatible with the rules of the Arizona State Board of Nursing. We also anticipate exploring a multiskilled clerical worker role that could combine some unit secretary, admissions, medical records, and utilization management functions.

Patient-focused care with less fragmentation is the goal. Our first steps have resulted in positive outcomes. Increased efficiency, effectiveness, and customer satisfaction have been demonstrated. We are encouraged that further efforts will enhance our outcomes and delight our customers.

REFERENCES

Alexander, J. (1992, May). *Operational restructuring: 19 pioneering models.* Paper presented at the Healthcare Forum Executive Conference, Ann Arbor, MI.

Bernd, D. L. (1992, December). Patient-focused care pays hospital-wide dividends. COO interview. *Health Care Strategic Management, 10,* 9-12.

Bernd, D. L., Kern, H. P., & Wharton, S. (1993, March). *Patient-focused hospital leadership strategy: A formula for success. Sentara Health System.* Paper presented at the Healthcare Forum Executive Conference, Pasadena, CA.

Drucker, P. (1992, February 11). Writing on teams. *Wall Street Journal.*

Farris, B. J., & O'Day, L. (1993, March). *Care 2001: Leading the way. St. Vincent Hospital and Health Care Center, Inc.* Paper presented at the Healthcare Forum Executive Conference, Pasadena, CA.

Feutz-Hartz, S. A. (1988). Nursing work assignment: Rights and responsibilities. *Journal of Nursing Administration, 18*(4), 9-11.

Johnson, W., & Miller, K. (1992). Strategies for healthcare excellence: Case study. *Organizational Productivity, Quality, and Effectiveness, 5*(10), 1-12.

Kohles, M. K., & Donaho, B. A. (1992). Patient-centered care. *Strategies for Healthcare Excellence, 5*(11), 1-12.

Lathrop, J. P. (1993, March). *The patient-focused hospital.* Paper presented at the Healthcare Forum Executive Conference, Pasadena, CA.

Leander, W. (1992, Spring). Dimensions of successful service redeployment: Why "service redeployment" succeeds where "department decentralization" fails. *PFCA Review,* pp. 2-7.

Lee, J. G., & Clarke, R. W. (1992, November). Restructuring improves hospital competitiveness. *Healthcare Financial Management, 46,* 30-37.

Murphy, E. C. (1992). How healthcare-specific quality initiatives impact the bottom line. *Organizational Productivity, Quality, and Effectiveness, 5*(10), 9-12.

National Council of State Boards of Nursing, Inc. (1987, August). *Statement on the Nursing Activities of Unlicensed Persons.* Reproduced in the booklet of the Satellite Teleconference of the American Hospital Association: Delegating Tasks to Nurse Assistive Personnel: Methods and Legal Responsibilities, September 1989.

Ritter, J., & Tonges, M. C. (1991). Work redesign in high-intensity environments: ProACT for critical care. *Journal of Nursing Administration, 21*(21), 26-34.

Stephens, J. R., Jones, D. T., & Watson, P. M. (1993, March). *Pioneering patient-focused care. Lakeland Regional Medical Center.* Paper presented at the Healthcare Forum Executive Conference, Pasadena, CA.

Tonges, M. C. (1989a). Redesigning hospital nursing practice: The professionally advanced care team (ProACT^{TM}) Model, Part 1. *Journal of Nursing Administration, 19*(7), 32-38.

Tonges, M. C. (1989b). Redesigning hospital nursing practice: The professionally advanced care team (ProACT^{TM}) Model, Part 2. *Journal of Nursing Administration, 19*(9), 19-22.

Urmy, N. B., Dubree, M. A., & Spinella, J. L. (1993, March). *Collaborative work redesign: Improving patient care and employee jobs. Vanderbilt University Hospital and Clinic.* Paper presented at the Healthcare Forum Executive Conference, Pasadena, CA.

Yarbrough, M. G., Tornabeni, J., & Scott, M. (1993, March). *Creating a culture to succeed. Mercy Hospital and Medical Center.* Paper presented at the Healthcare Forum Executive Conference, Pasadena, CA.

Zimmerman, J., Crosier, J., & Taylor, S. (1993, Winter). Support service assistants: Redesigning roles for patient-centered care. *Stanford Nurse, 15,* 3-6.

CHAPTER 9

Implementation and Evaluation of Patient-Centered Care

Katherine R. Jones
Vicki DeBaca
Jolene Tornebeni
Mary Yarbrough

Health care organizations are being restructured and redesigned in order to provide exceptional customer service and quality of care while improving efficiency and productivity in care delivery. One approach is called Patient-Focused Care, and involves integration of services and caregivers around the needs of the primary hospital customer, the patient. After an extensive evaluation of internal and external customers' needs and expectations, Mercy Health Care of San Diego, California, implemented the Patient-Focused Care Model of service delivery. Components of the model include decentralizing services to the unit or patient room when possible, creating multiskilled workers through cross-training, and using bedside computers with exceptions documentation. Caregivers, physicians, and patients have participated in the evaluation of the new system, and information on work allocation and quality of care has also been collected. Analyses indicate that positive results are being achieved, supporting the extension of the model to additional units in the hospital. This chapter discusses the advantages and problems associated with the implementation of the Patient-Focused Care Model at one medical center. It presents lessons learned that might be helpful to others as they implement this or other complex but innovative approaches to restructuring.

Health care executives in general, and nurse executives in particular, have a professional responsibility to design delivery systems that ensure high-quality care and financial viability (Robinson, 1991). Organizational restructuring and work redesign strategies have been developed in response to several identified problems in today's hospitals (Borzo, 1992):

1. Many employees have become functional specialists who perform limited, repetitive tasks.
2. Hospitals have become compartmentalized, resulting in fragmented, impersonal care.
3. Much professional time is spent documenting work, being "ready for work" (but waiting for information, orders, or other personnel), scheduling activities, and coordinating care delivery systems rather than providing and managing direct patient care.
4. Multiple process steps are required for each ordered activity, with excessive patient contacts by different caregivers.

The results of the above problems include narrowly defined roles, with allegiance to departments rather than to patients; much time consumed in activities or waiting periods that contribute little to the value of the services received by patients; and much time spent by patients in transit to various appointments and interacting with a vast array of different caregivers, most of whom are unknown to them. It is apparent that substantial changes are necessary in the organization and delivery of services in hospitals to improve both efficiency and productivity.

A restructuring approach that addresses the described problem areas is called the Patient-Focused Care Model. In this model, the patient provides the focus for integrating all services provided by the institution. Staff and services are organized around the needs of patients, rather than departments or disciplines, and emphasis is placed on meeting individualized patient care needs. There are three key components to a patient-focused hospital: (a) Staff is cross-trained, and teams of multiskilled caregivers are created; (b) services such as pharmacy and admitting are decentralized and moved to patient rooms or the patient care unit whenever possible; and (c) protocols of care and computerized exception-reporting medical records are established.

The organization embarking on such a major redesign effort needs to develop and implement a comprehensive evaluation plan to monitor the implementation and impact of the new roles and structures. This chapter presents selected results of a systematic plan to evaluate the transition to this model in one medical center. It focuses on several key elements of the model, and traces their evolution over the 2-year implementation period. The chapter concludes with a summary of the advantages and disadvantages of this model, and strategies for overcoming potential barriers to this innovative approach to restructuring.

DATA-BASED PLANNING

Focus Groups

The essential initial step to substantive restructuring is an organizational commitment to change the environment based on the needs and wants of the customers. Customer service has become the most important base of competition in today's health care marketplace (O'Malley & Serpico-Thompson, 1992). The most frequently identified, and arguably the most important, customers of hospitals are patients. The goal of the organizational restructuring and role redesign efforts described in this chapter was to create a patient-focused environment that would enhance patient satisfaction and perception of quality of the service experience. Other customers within the hospital include physicians, employees, and vendors, all of whom are brought together to provide services and products to patients in the health care setting.

As the first step in the institution's restructuring program, focus groups were conducted to determine the expectations of the primary customer, the patients. The intent was to determine what would enhance the patients' perceptions of quality and overall satisfaction. A sample of subjects was recruited from the local geographic area by an independent focus survey company. Recruited participants were unaware of the sponsoring institution. Participants included those who had been previous patients of the institution, those who had received care at other hospitals within the geographic area, and those who had no hospital experience.

The focus groups were conducted by an experienced, professional interviewer. A semistructured interview guide was used to gather information in the following areas: likes and dislikes relating to past hospital experiences; expectations during the hospital experience; identification of ideal hospital experiences; and suggestions for improvements in the current hospital environment. Focus group participants said that they wanted a caring and concerned staff who were also competent in carrying out their responsibilities; clear and consistent communication with the physician and hospital personnel; a quiet and clean environment; more choices in terms of services and routines; and less waiting, especially during admission and discharge from the hospital. The patients also made several innovative suggestions for improved services. They made the recommendation that one person be designated as the official "communicator" with patients, to avoid the problem of inconsistent and conflicting messages from different personnel. They requested follow-up phone calls at home after discharge, as well as business cards from primary nurses and other relevant caregivers to facilitate continuity of care.

Employee focus groups were next conducted, in which the expectations and concerns of past and potential customers were shared with those who were responsible for the actual point-of-service delivery of care at the institution. A group of hospital employees representing all departments, job categories (except physicians), and working shifts was invited to participate in employee focus groups. The purpose of these groups was to share feedback about patient expectations and to make recommendations about how the structure and processes of the organization could be redesigned to more effectively meet patients' needs and expectations.

A semistructured interview questionnaire and an independent consultant were again used to gather information that was to provide a foundation for the redesign effort. Suggestions for improvement made by these focus group participants could be classified as procedural and structural recommendations for change. These included the desire for more staff, better understanding and communication between departments, more information sharing within the organization, beepers/pagers for caregivers, more assistance with non-English-speaking patients, and better access to supplies, equipment, and other resources for patient care.

Work Sampling

Work sampling by the Industrial Engineering Department revealed the extent of compartmentalization within the organization. Compartmentalization reflects a highly specialized and fragmented organization (Watson, Shortridge, Jones, Rees, & Stephens, 1991). The largest single blocks of time were being spent on patient care documentation and being "ready for work," and a lesser amount of time was being spent on the delivery of direct patient care. The inefficiencies associated with compartmentalization include volatile workloads and structured idle time, limited flexibility to accommodate change, complex interdepartmental relationships, and high costs of coordination, scheduling, documenting, and managing care processes (Watson et al., 1991).

RESTRUCTURING FOR PATIENT-FOCUSED CARE

Planning

In order to ensure extensive participation and communication within the complex organizational structure, a team committee structure was developed that included a broad representation of employees. There were three levels to the project team. At the core was a Steering Committee, consisting of senior management, physicians, patient care directors, and representatives from Human Resources, Facilities, Information Systems, and Finance. The responsibilities of the Steering Committee included development and communication of the project vision, resource allocation, financial decisions, guidance and support to other team members, and championing of the overall project. At the next level was the Team Leader Committee, which was composed of the staff and managers or supervisors representing all departments that came into contact with the patients. This committee met weekly to define roles, create facility redesign, and develop systems and protocols for the functioning of patient-focused units. Eleven other committees and task forces had more focused spheres of concerns: information systems, legal aspects, phone support, facility and equipment, training, documentation, human resources, quality assurance, transition, activation, and communication. These committees worked closely with the Team Leader Committee to fashion structures and processes that addressed the major concerns of the internal and external customers.

WORK REDESIGN

The operating principles for the organizational restructuring and role redesign were to (a) streamline documentation requirements, (b) place patient services closer to the patient, (c) simplify work processes, (d) focus patient populations in specific geographic areas and develop scale, and (e) broaden caregiver qualifications. The key components of the selected model are cross-training of personnel to achieve multiskilled workers; decentralization of services to patient care units and room whenever possible; and use of computerized exception reporting with bedside computers. The multiskilled workers are prepared at four levels: clinical, technical, service, and administrative. The clinical partner is a licensed staff member such as an RN, pharmacist, or medical technologist. The clinical care components involve bedside care, rehabilitative therapies, specific diagnostic procedures, and pharmacy. The technical partner is someone with previous patient care experience, such as an LVN or a physical therapy technician. He or she assists the clinical partner in carrying out patient care activities. The service partner carries out the support functions of housekeeping, stocking patient servers, materials management, transportation of patients and supplies, visitor reception, errands, and meal delivery. The administrative partner carries out secretarial, receptionist, and medical records responsibilities, including admitting and discharge procedures, coding and abstracting medical records, and scheduling activities.

Patient care assignments are made to "care pairs" consisting of two clinical partners or a clinic partner and technical partner. Care pairs attend to six to eight patients on a given unit and work 12-hour shifts together. The pairing of partners is flexible, to better meet the specific patient care requirements. However, one clinical partner is always a registered nurse. Each partner carries a pager that is programmed to the assigned patients' rooms. This facilitates communication and coordination of activities between the pair, and between the pair and the central desk.

A core curriculum, developed and taught by staff educators and clinical nurse specialists, includes didactic sessions, skill practice laboratories, preceptorships, and transitional support groups. The core curriculum reflects a foundation of basic skills that are common to all partner categories. These include bed making, vital sign measurement, and patient positioning. Additional classes are targeted for caregivers on specific units (for example, total hip and knee care for the orthopedic unit staff only); others are limited to specific caregiver categories, such as financial procedures for the administrative partners only.

The selected work redesign strategy was implemented on two pilot units, and two other units served as controls during the implementation and evaluation process. The two pilot units were selected for introduction of the model based on two sets of consideration. One unit had well-defined, clearly understood work processes, had an interested and motivated manager and staff, and was typically a unit on which this model was introduced in other settings. The second pilot unit had less well-defined work processes and procedures, and a less enthusiastic staff and manager. It was felt that this input provided an ideal opportunity for improvement in care delivery processes and would be a good test of the model's ability to improve work effectiveness and efficiency in less than ideal circumstances.

Reducing Patient Waiting Times

One strategy to reduce the amount of time patients spent traveling to appointments, being admitted, or waiting for specific services on the unit is to decentralize as many services as possible to the patient care unit or the patient's room. Decentralization initiatives have the potential to eliminate the 40% downtime that centralized departments spend going to and from patient care units, and also to integrate the service providers into a single team to allow focusing of services to the customer (Strasen, 1991). A serious delay always seemed to occur at time of patient admission to the hospital. Patients (and their families) would have to wait on average 15 or more minutes to be admitted to their room under the centralized system. Very often the patient was in pain or in some discomfort, and many times these admission waits would extend over mealtimes. Patients began their hospitalization experiences tired of waiting, hungry, and frustrated with hospital "routines." The restructured environment provides for patient admission directly to the patient care unit. There is a patient reception area on each redesigned unit, where one of the administrative partners carries out the admitting routines. The time required to admit a patient to his or her room has been reduced to 5 minutes.

Another useful strategy for reducing patient and staff waiting times is the introduction of bedside "patient servers." Patient servers contain the patient chart, medications, and supplies specific to the patient's needs. This medication availability reduces the time required to prepare and administer medications, particularly pain medication. This also reduces the amount of steps required by the nurse to determine patient needs, retrieve the requisite medication, and return to the patient's room to administer the drug. Patient servers also contain linen and other supplies, again reducing the amount of walking required of the caregivers.

Patient and staff transportation and waiting times are also reduced through the decentralizing of clinical services to the unit, particularly pharmacy and laboratory services, which simplifies ordering and scheduling processes. Having these services and this type of personnel readily available on the patient care units switches the focus from the separate departments to individual patient care needs.

For example, staff no longer have to call for a phlebotomist when a blood test is ordered for the patient. The floor-based phlebotomist or multiskilled worker can draw the blood specimen, and the simple procedures can be analyzed in the unit-based laboratory. Laboratory test reporting is done with very quick turnaround times. The costs of having a unit-based laboratory are offset by having fewer FTEs and less equipment in the central laboratory.

Pharmacists and pharmacy technicians are also located on the patient care units and are available to meet patient care needs on a continuous basis. New units have pharmacies open 12 hours a day. Automated narcotic-dispensing machines and locked medicine drawers in patient rooms allow access to medications around the clock. Pharmacists are able to work closely with physicians in determining optimal therapeutic regimens, and also with other caregivers and the patients to monitor responses to the introduction of new therapies or to alterations in existing therapies. Having key patient-related services on the units improves responsiveness to physician needs, promotes continuity of care, reduces patient time spent off the unit, and minimizes transportation and documentation requirements.

Reducing Multiple Contacts

One of the problem areas identified in the literature and by the focus groups was multiple patient contacts by multiple caregivers within the hospital. These contacts tended to be truncated and impersonal, as well as task oriented and not patient focused. One way to improve this situation is to carry out cross-training of all levels of personnel, which broadens caregiver qualifications. Multidisciplinary caregiver teams bring together individuals from different disciplines with different perspectives for one single reason—to provide high-quality care to patients. The team strives to get beyond disciplinary and departmental allegiances to achieve open communication, camaraderie, and loyalty among team members (Donaho & Kohles, 1992). Support staff, administrative personnel, technical staff, and professional personnel all underwent a series of training sessions with the purpose of producing multiskilled workers, with the overall goal being to enhance the sensitivity of all categories of personnel to patient needs and wants.

Rather than having multiple types of caregivers, each of whom performs one or two tasks for any particular patient, there are a limited number of caregiver types, each able to perform a wider variety of tasks for the individual patient. Most important, the cross-training efforts provides a larger cadre of personnel who respond to basic patient concerns. The patient is less likely to hear, "That's not my job."

Cross-Training Issues

Several issues had to be resolved relating to the cross-training of personnel, for example, which skills needed to be included in the various multiskilled caregiver roles. It was decided that all clinical and technical partners were to be prepared to give basic patient care, as well as to do specific technical procedures. Some skills considered for cross-training needed special arrangements or were omitted because of legal considerations. Specifically, a matrix reporting relationship was established for the medical technologists, who could not report solely to a nursing unit director. Instead, the medical technologists report to the unit director for operational issues, and to the director of the clinical laboratory for professional/technical issues. This arrangement ensures that the medical technologist remains up to date professionally with advances in laboratory procedures and technologies, but also remains integrated with the patient care focus on the unit. Radiology procedures, on the other hand, were not decentralized to the patient care units because of state regulations requiring radiology technicians to function under the direct supervision of a radiologist.

Feedback from the preceptors led to a conclusion that the initial training period was of insufficient duration to ensure competency and confidence in many of the newly acquired skills. The cross-trained individuals were insecure and hesitant to carry out their new job responsibilities. The training period was extended by 1 week, allowing for more practice time. Preceptors reported that cross-trained individuals appeared more secure and that transition on the units to the newly defined caregiver roles was proceeding more smoothly. These competency evaluations were accomplished using several different approaches. One was the direct observation of caregivers by the assigned preceptors. Unit directors also observed performance levels and provided feedback to the educators and clinical nurse specialists. In addition, ancillary departments developed specific evaluation protocols. For example, medical personnel from cardiology conducted analyses of EKG performance by comparing tracings done by cross-trained individuals to objective performance criteria, as well as comparing the accuracy and proficiency of cross-trained individuals to that of cardiology personnel doing EKG tracing.

Patient-Focused Care: Evaluation

Work evaluation. Donaho and Kohles (1992) believe that a certain level of tension occurs when cross-trained workers are introduced onto units and skill mixes begin to change. Some of the routine tasks traditionally done by nurses are now carried out by the multiskilled worker, so the nurses must learn to delegate and "let go" of some of the traditional tasks. Work sampling was carried out to determine how caregiver time was actually being distributed across the various role components after the cross-training sessions and implementation of the Patient-Focused Care Model. Caregivers were followed and their activities recorded by nonparticipant observers from the Industrial Engineering Department, who noted time spent performing tasks in the major subcategories of work (patient documentation, transportation, and so on). Results indicated that differences existed across caregiver partner category and by whether the caregiver was on a unit that had implemented the Patient-Focused Care Model (a pilot unit) or had remained with the traditional delivery system (a control unit). On one of the pilot units, it was discovered that the pharmacist's clinical partner was confining his/her activities to only two realms, medical/technical services (80%) and scheduling (20%), and ignoring the other patient care activities that were part of the multiskilled role. In contrast, the pharmacist on the other pilot unit allocated work time across multiple activities, including medical/technical (26%), supply transport (23%), medical documentation (17%), being out of area (15%), scheduling (10%), and hotel services (5%). Further analysis of the pharmacist role revealed that on the first unit, the pharmacist had taken advantage of the patient unit placement to expand the pharmacist's role in terms of patient drug education and monitoring, consulting with physicians, and checking medication orders for dosages, incompatibilities, and so on, rather than performing "nonpharmacist" activities. Although this was not the intent of the caregiver role redesign, it has led to discussions as to whether such differences in role implementation may be more beneficial to patient outcomes than a rigid adherence to the true intent of the role redesign.

Interestingly, the administrative partner and service partner roles showed more evidence of the desired multiskilling on the first unit than on the second pilot unit. On the first unit, administrative partners divided their time among scheduling (36%), documentation (24%), supply transport (14%), technical activities (10%), hotel services (6%), being out of area (5%), and transporting (3%), whereas on the second unit administrative partners did medical documentation (59%) primarily, with scheduling (14%) and being out of area (15%) taking up most of the rest of their time. Service partner differences were also striking: On the first unit they spent time doing hotel services (34%), transporting supplies (22%), technical activities (12%), scheduling (9%), being out of area (9%), and documenting (8%), whereas on the second unit the service partners spent 92% of their time on hotel services, with 6% allocated to supply transport and 3% to being out of area.

The RN role was the most consistent across the two units. RNs on both pilot units spent the greatest amount of their time on medical/technical services (46% and 37%), followed by documentation (17% and 20%) and scheduling (8% and 15%). They also supervised (8% and 2%), provided hotel services (6% and 5%), transported supplies (5% and 13%), were "ready for care" (5% and 2%), and were out of the area (7% and 4%). Analyses in late 1990 showed that nurses at that time spent only 30% of their time in direct patient care activities, as compared to the 46% and 37% shown above, so progress toward one desired outcome is being made.

Overall evaluation of how time was spent on the various activities before and after implementation of patient-focused care revealed both desired and unexpected findings. On the positive side, one of the pilot units showed a 12% increase in the amount of time spent on medical/technical activities, but it also experienced a 5% increase in patient documentation, which was not desired. At the same time, there were the desired decreases in the amount of time spent in institutional documentation and supply transport. The second pilot unit, however, showed no increase in the time spent on medical/technical services, and a substantial increase (8% to 20%) in the time spent on patient documentation. On the positive side, this unit also experienced a decrease in amount of time spent on supervision, being ready for care, and being out of area. Interestingly, one of the control units demonstrated the desired increase in the amount of time spent on medical/technical services, as well as a decrease in the time spent on patient documentation and supply transport.

Caregiver Evaluation. A comprehensive caregiver survey packet was developed by the senior author (Katherine R. Jones) in collaboration with the coauthors and other key individuals at Mercy Health Care System. The instruments were pilot tested by members of the Steering and Team Leader Committees, revised, and then distributed to individuals whose job categories fell within one of the cross-trained caregiver categories. Surveys were completed approximately 3 months before implementation of the Patient-Focused Care Model, and again approximately 9 months after implementation of the model on the two selected pilot units. The instruments included in the survey packet measured organizational culture, work group processes, staff attitudes toward work flow and change, communication, and satisfaction. Reliability testing of the instruments elicited Cronbach's alpha scores for internal consistency that were all in the moderate to strong ranges.

Attitudes Toward Work Flow and Change. The questions relating to work flow and changed health dealt primarily with interdepartmental and interprofessional relationships, and with resistance to the changes introduced by the patient-focused care model. The pilot units together did not achieve the most positive scores for improved work flow between departments and disciplines. Instead, one of the pilot units appeared to experience difficulty in the transition to the new model and actually achieved lower scores than one of the control units. These lower scores were also seen on the communication survey and satisfaction survey. These findings were supported by anecdotal evidence and observations by the project leader and other key personnel. To facilitate the transition to patient-focused care on this unit, special sessions were held with the human resource coordinators, and team-building activities were carried out.

Among the different caregiver categories, survey results indicated that the clerical staff and the support staff had statistically more significant positive responses on the work flow items than the RN, other professional, and technical caregiver categories. The support staff group and other professional group, on the other hand, had the most positive responses on the items relating to changes occurring in the environment. But these were not statistically different from the responses of the other caregiver categories.

Work Group Processes. Another section of the caregiver surveys described perceptions of work group effectiveness. This survey incorporated items from an instrument developed at Vanderbilt University Hospital to help evaluate their Strengthening Hospital Performance grant, and also had other items that were specific to the Mercy Hospital experience. The major constructs measured in the instrument were work group stability, preference for the status quo, goal clarity, group commitment, group cohesiveness, group productivity, and environmental support. Although basic perceptions of work group effectiveness did not change significantly between baseline and postimplementation periods, there were interesting subgroup differences. The support staff showed a substantial increase in perceived work group stability after implementing the new model and perceived significantly higher stability than the other caregiver categories. This group also demonstrated substantial increases in their perceived work group clarity, work group commitment, and work group cohesiveness scores post implementation. Conversely, the other professional group (pharmacists, medical technologists) experienced a decrease in their group commitment and group cohesiveness scores, reflecting less satisfaction with work group processes in the postimplementation period. All caregiver groups perceived lower environmental support for the work group after implementation of patient-focused care. The only significant difference across the patient care units was that one of the control units had a significantly higher mean score on preference for the status quo. This and other information factored into plans for the second phase of implementation of patient-focused care within the hospital.

Job Satisfaction

The major intent of role redesign is to create roles that increase job satisfaction and performance (Tumulty, 1992). However, caregiver satisfaction scores displayed little change between the two data collection periods. It was gratifying to see that the few increases in level of satisfaction were on those items relating to patient care: satisfaction with the care people receive at the hospital; satisfaction with the care people receive on the unit; and satisfaction with patient-caregiver relationships. The least amount of satisfaction was expressed with salary, fringe benefits, recognition, and staffing levels, and the highest amount of satisfaction was expressed for people in the work group, the type of work, and work group performance. Subgroup analysis revealed that there were no significant differences in level of satisfaction across the different caregiver categories, but that the other professional group and the support staff group had greater satisfaction with interpersonal relationships after implementation of patient-focused care, whereas the clerical staff had less satisfaction with aspects of the work group itself.

Organizational Communication. The communication survey in the caregiver evaluation packet was the nine-item organization communication assessment developed by Farley (1989). The least positive responses were obtained on items relating to perceived effectiveness of administration's communication with employees; administration's sharing of critical and pertinent information with employees; and receipt of information about what is going on in the hospital. These remained essentially unchanged between the two survey periods. However, caregiver satisfaction with frequency of communication with the supervisor declined in the postimplementation period, although the level of satisfaction with communication with one's supervisor was higher than the level of satisfaction with communication with hospital administration.

Medical Staff Evaluation

Another important customer of the hospital is the medical staff. Physicians have a choice of where to admit their patients, so they must have a high level of satisfaction with the quality of care delivered to their patients in any particular setting. Consequently we set out to assess their perceptions of care delivery and their reactions to how the newly restructured system and redefined caregiver roles affected their patients.

A short, 25-item survey was developed by the lead author, in collaboration with key individuals at the Mercy Health Care System, and mailed to physicians with admitting privileges at the Medical Center before and after implementation of patient-focused care. It was completed and returned by 29 physicians in the preimplementation period and 31 physicians in the postimplementation period.

Almost all of the responses increased in the postimplementation period, indicating a higher level of satisfaction with the care being delivered on the units. The greatest amount of satisfaction was expressed for the following items: caregivers treat me courteously, adequate precautions are taken to prevent patient injuries, caregivers are competent in carrying out their duties, supplies and equipment are in good condition, and caregivers give me accurate information about my patients. Physicians expressed the least amount of satisfaction with the following items: I can find a caregiver quickly when I am on the units, the staffing level seems adequate, caregivers are available when I need assistance, caregivers have time to care properly for my patients, and caregivers are able to solve problems that occur on the unit. The greatest increase in level of satisfaction that occurred between the two data collection periods was for the following items: Patients' rooms are neat and orderly, caregivers have time to care properly for my patients, caregivers are competent when carrying out their duties, caregivers attend to my patients' emotional needs, families are supplied with adequate information, and the staffing level seems adequate. None of the decreases in mean level of satisfaction on specific items on the survey were statistically significant.

Responses by physicians to a question on overall quality of care delivered to their patients over the past 2 weeks also demonstrated improvement after implementation of patient-focused care. In the preimplementation period, no physicians described the care as excellent, 29% said it was very good, 54% said it was satisfactory, and 14% said it was only fair. In comparison, 14% of the physicians described the care as excellent in the postimplementation period, with another 41% saying that it was very good. In addition, 31% described it as satisfactory, 10% as only fair, and 4% as unsatisfactory.

A follow-up survey done on a smaller number of physicians from the pilot units revealed more specific likes and dislikes about the newly implemented structure. Physicians commented that the quality of care had significantly improved, that the nursing "partners" were very helpful, that their patients liked the new system better, that laboratory results were returned very quickly, and that they perceived that the nurses felt more accountable for care delivered on the units. The physicians, however, did not like standing at the bedside computer, and felt that they needed space away from the patient to review the chart and discuss the patient's condition. They also felt that the telephones were a problem and that the system was not very efficient. More specifically, it was sometimes difficult to get the telephone answered on the pilot units, and if it was answered, there was sometimes a lengthy delay before the appropriate caregiver came to the telephone. This problem was resolved by the pocket paging system so that the appropriate caregivers were immediately informed on incoming telephoning calls. The majority of the physician respondents indicated that they would not want to see a return to the "old" way of doing things.

Patient Evaluation

Patient care directors who make regular rounds to patients report anecdotally that the number of patient concerns has decreased for those hospitalized on the restructured units. The patients report more satisfaction with the visibility of caregivers, and the more frequent contact with caregivers results in improved communication with patients and their families. These factors have combined to improve the patients' perceptions about the quality of care being provided.

More objective data collected through patient satisfaction surveys developed by Press-Ganey and distributed by the hospital on a regular basis also indicate a positive trend toward greater patient satisfaction on the pilot units. One pilot unit's average satisfaction scores increased from 84.8 to 89.4 after implementation of patient-focused care; the other pilot unit's average satisfaction scores increased from 81.4 to 85.4. There was no increase in average patient satisfaction scores for the institution as a whole. On one of these units, three of the four quarters in 1992 (post implementation) had higher average patient satisfaction scores than achieved in any quarter in 1991.

There are also indications that quality of care has improved on the pilot units. Patient falls on the second pilot unit have been reduced by approximately 50%. Infection rates on the unit have been reduced in the three primary categories of urinary tract, bloodstream, and pneumonia. In addition, service time for patient registration and laboratory tests has been significantly reduced on both pilot units.

LESSONS LEARNED

There are many potential benefits of patient-focused care. These include improved caregiver effectiveness, reduced response times, reduced length of stay, increased efficiency and flexibility, and more satisfied frontline work groups and customers. These and other items should be monitored on a continuous basis to ensure successful achievement and continuous improvement of these positive outcomes. Selected results of one hospital's experience in adopting this new organizational model have been presented. A primary lesson learned in the described transition to a patient-focused model of care delivery is the importance of communication. The most negative responses on the physician and caregiver surveys related to level of communication about the changes taking place in the hospital. People never seemed to feel that they had received enough information about changes that affected their jobs and the way things were done in their work setting. The caregiver surveys revealed increasing concern about extent and clarity of communication as one moved from peer group communication to communication with middle management and then to communication with upper management. Information must be conveyed from upper administrative levels in the organization to all involved stockholders on a consistent and continuous basis. Information must be transmitted by as many routes as possible, and it must be repeated as often as possible. Communication channels need to include retreats, departmental and unit meetings, interdepartmental meetings, newsletters, written and verbal feedback on results being attained, and one-on-one interactions.

There is also a need to constantly reinforce new learning and to pay attention to the changes taking place in the organization. It is very easy to slip back into the "old ways" of doing things because these have a higher comfort level than the new ways. There must be continuous measurement of the outcomes of the restructuring, both to facilitate celebration of accomplishments and to detect and correct problems in the newly restructured roles and responsibilities.

Perhaps most important is the need to hold people accountable. The various employee groups were deeply involved with the development and operationalization of the model, which represented one component of the organization's stated 21st-Century themes: continuous quality improvement, shared governance, and patient-focused care. Staff empowerment is achieved through the strong tradition of shared governance at Mercy Health Care System. Extensive staff participation throughout the entire organizational restructuring process contributed to a sense of ownership and staff buy-in to the newly implemented model of care. This facilitated the commitment of various employee groups to their new roles, behaviors, and reporting relationships. However, certain groups of staff were more ready for implementation of the model than others, which led to some implementation problems and additional change strategies.

The focus on customer service and the opportunity to improve the services being delivered to the customers fit well within the continuous quality improvement model. The goal is the achievement of a continual state of improvement in patient and organizational outcomes, within the necessary cost constraints. Organizational change and renewal never reaches a final stage, but rather continues to evolve into new structures and roles that promote ever-increasing levels of effectiveness and efficiency.

The Patient-Focused Care Model is not inexpensive to implement. The physical reconfiguration of the patient care units requires construction dollars, and the time requirements for cross-training (instructor, preceptor, and learner time) are substantial. In addition, there are consultant and capital equipment costs. However, once a critical mass of units and individuals are functioning under the new model, FTEs in the ancillary departments are reduced. For example, now that four patient units have implemented patient-focused care, 100 FTEs have been omitted from the pharmacy, laboratory, central services, and food services departments, and further reductions will occur. There are also cost savings from the productivity and work process improvement.

The patient-focused model of care delivery can serve to strengthen professional nursing practice. The presence of multiskilled workers and the utilization of care pairs frees the nurse from performing nonessential tasks because the tasks can now be delegated to the technical or service partners on the units. This delegation provides time for performing the higher level functions of patient and family teaching and discharge planning. The nurse also spends more time in care management, both planning and coordinating the care required by patients. The successful provision of coordinated care serves to promote both effectiveness in terms of positive outcomes and efficiency in terms of timely discharge from the hospital.

In addition, the Patient-Focused Care Model brings added value to the bedside. A larger number of individuals are available on the unit to respond to patient and family needs and requests. A larger number of services are available on the unit, decreasing the time the patient spends in transit and receiving services at remote sites.

The Patient-Focused Care Model described in this chapter represents an institutional, not nursing, model of care, as recommended by Fralic (1992). Implementation of the model was based on a systematic analysis of the work of patient care delivery on each unit, with subsequent restructuring of the work and redesigning of new roles. Ongoing feedback during the implementation phase led to refinements in the training process and to special sessions with the human resource coordinator for team building and values clarification.

Additional analyses are being carried out that will document the continuing influence of the restructured system of care delivery on specific quality indicators and costs. Evidence has been examined that indicates that lengths of stay on the pilot units have been reduced as a result of the new care delivery model. All indicators thus far suggest that the patient-focused model of care is a feasible option for health care organizations facing uncertain futures and requiring substantial changes in how the work gets done.

REFERENCES

Borzo, G. (1992). Patient-focused hospitals begin reporting good results. *Human Resources Strategic Management, 10*(8),1, 17-22.

Donaho, B., & Kohles, M. K. (1992). Multi-disciplinary caregiver teams: Key to patient-centered care. *Strengthening, 1*(1), 1-8.

Farley, M. J. (1989). Assessing communication in organizations. *Journal of Nursing Administration, 19*(12), 27-31.

Fralic, M. F. (1992). Creating new practice models and designing new roles: Reflections and recommendations. *Journal of Nursing Administration, 22*(6), 7-8.

O'Malley, J., & Serpico-Thompson, D. (1992). Redesigning roles for patient-centered care: The hospitality representative. *Journal of Nursing Administration, 22*(7/8), 30-34.

Robinson, N. C. (1991). A patient-centered framework for restructuring care. *Journal of Nursing Administration, 21*(9), 29-34.

Strasen, L. (1991). Redesigning hospitals around patients and technology. *Nursing Economics, 9*(4), 233-238.

Tumulty, G. (1992). Head nurse role redesign: Improving satisfaction and performance. *Journal of Nursing Administration, 22*(2), 41-48.

Watson, P. M., Shortridge, D. L., Jones, D. T., Rees, R. T., & Stephens, J. T. (1991). Organizational restructuring: A patient-focused approach. *Nursing Administration Quarterly, 16*(1), 45-52.

CHAPTER 10

The Community Design Model: A Framework for Restructuring

Paula Siler
Maryalice Jordan-Marsh
Peggy Nazarey
Susan R. Goldsmith
Elisa Sanchez

Restructuring begins at the organizational level with reengineering and moves to the service level with work redesign. An organizational design model is a framework for restructuring. The Community Design Model is presented as a prototype for responding to and managing broad-scale organizational change. The model has four key components: a conceptual framework, strategic directions, outcome indicators, and strategic management processes. Application of the model is described in terms of the work in progress in one academic medical center. Achievements and lessons learned will be addressed under the outcome indicators: culture, structures, systems, and learning/competence.

Earlier definitions of work redesign focused on the structure of the job and altering specific jobs (or interdependent systems of jobs) to improve productivity and quality of work life (Hackman, 1980, cited in Tonges, 1992). Recently, there has been a paradigm shift in contemporary work redesign literature. The focus now is on the outcome of the job or work as it affects the customer. Reengineering (Hammer & Champy, 1993) combined with work redesign captures this goal of a customer-oriented perspective. In health care, the primary customer is the patient and family. Customers can also be internal, such as nurses and physicians, or external, such as vendors and payers. The challenge is to define the mission of the organization to include the interest and concerns of all customers holding a stake in its future (stakeholders).

A second focus is on changes in the specifics of the work and or unit operations to a model for organization-wide change. Reengineering requires both changes in relationships and resources and the ability to conceptualize the whole without dividing work into tasks (Liu, Denis, Kolodny, & Stymne, 1990).

Organizational restructuring calls for both reengineeering and work re-design. The result maximizes both social and technical aspects of work. Re-structuring can be as simple as flexing to allow for autonomy and variation within a single work unit such as pediatrics (work redesign), or it may be as complex as total redesign of the way work is accomplished across the organization (reengineering).

This chapter will present a model for restructuring that begins at the organizational level with reengineering and moves to the service level with work redesign. The service level is the interface between the customer and the work. Elements central to the goal of reengineering will be outlined. Related work redesign will be described under the application section. The description of our application will begin with a historical perspective. Progress toward achievement of outcomes of quality patient care, a quality work life, and organizational effectiveness will be addressed in terms of the community design model (CDM) outcome indicators. Changes at the organizational and service levels will be highlighted.

ELEMENTS OF REENGINEERING

Reengineering means a new beginning and starting over to ask not how we do things better, but why do we do what we do. Therefore, Hammer and Champy (1993) propose that broad-scale organizational change does not build from *kaizen* (Imai, 1986), the continuous incremental improvement of existing processes, but rather from a search for a new understanding of the work to be done. The concept of reengineering has been defined as "the fundamental rethinking and radical redesign of business processes to achieve dramatic improvement in critical, contemporary measures of performance, such as cost, quality and speed" (Hammer & Champy, 1993, p. 156). In this section, we will propose and describe a model for undertaking reengineering with application to a variety of settings. The model provides a basis for strategic management.

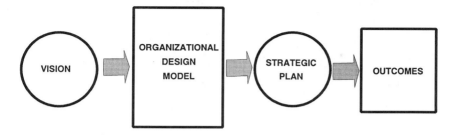

Figure 10.1. Components of a Reengineering Process

Starting Points

In order to conduct reengineering, the organization must embrace a vision of the future that identifies clear outcomes. A vision is essentially a dream that must be given voice and become grounded in reality (Helgesen, 1990). This reality gets shaped through an organizational design. Vision combined with design shapes the strategic plan, which determines the indicators of success in achieving the envisioned outcomes. "Vision provides a yardstick for measuring the progress of reengineering" (Hammer & Champy, 1993, p. 154).

Ideally, organizations create a vision of their future and adopt a specific organizational design model. Whatever the level of work redesign and/or organizational reengineering, the process is best achieved with a leadership group that articulates and communicates the vision, develops the strategic plan, and assumes oversight for strategic management.

An organizational design can then be selected or developed. An organizational design is a framework that identifies how people relate to each other, the organization, and the environment to accomplish common goals. The framework provides direction for a strategic plan shaped by the vision and values that characterize these relationships. An ideal organizational design specifies the outcomes it proposes to achieve, provides a conceptual framework and strategic directions, identifies outcome indicators to be addressed in the strategic plan and recommends processes for strategically managing the work (see Figure 10.1).

Hammer and Champy (1993) observe that

a lot of energy goes into designing organizations because the shape of the organization determines much about it, from how the company's work is organized to the mechanisms for the exercise of control and performance monitoring. The organizational structure establishes the lines of communication within the organization and determines the decision making hierarchy. (p. 78)

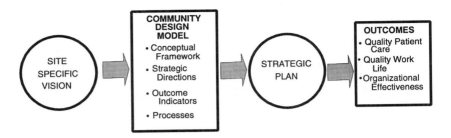

Figure 10.2. Proposal for the Reengineering Process Utilizing the Community
Design Model

An efficient organizational design will channel individual self-interests into
well-coordinated, socially productive activities that benefit the group (Milgrom,
1988). In this orientation, companies that have reengineered work become
organized around processes and self-directed work teams.

COMMUNITY DESIGN MODEL

The community design model (CDM) is an example of a framework for
broad-scale organizational change that is vision centered and has a conceptual
base. The purpose of the model is to assist organizations in the arduous process
of achieving their vision. The CDM has potential application in settings with
diverse visions. It is a framework for organizations whose goals are to achieve
vision-based, quality, customer-centered outcomes, a quality work life, and organizational effectiveness. The model has four key components: a conceptual
framework, strategic directions, outcome indicators, and strategic management processes, as reflected in Figure 10.2.

The model is responsive to the national interest in community. Renewed
interest in building a sense of community (Bellah, Madsen, Sullivan, Sidler, &
Tipton, 1985; Bennis, 1989; Covey, 1991) was given prominence in President
Clinton's inaugural address. Currently, there is a search for a way to shift from
the paradigm of "me" to "we" (Etzioni, 1993). As health care groups undertake
reforms to deal with the challenges of the 1990s and struggle with becoming
patient centered and worker sensitive, the concept of community has broad
appeal (Department of Nursing, 1990; Friedman, 1993). Community offers the
promise of bringing people together to achieve a common goal without com-
promising individual identity. People become recognized as the organization's

greatest resource. Development of their potential as leaders is the cornerstone of reengineering and work redesign in the CDM.

Conceptual Framework

The conceptual framework for the CDM is built on the assumption that success requires creating an internal sense of community, in combination with an expectation that every stakeholder (in health care—patients, faculty, staff, students, etc.) is a leader. The conceptual framework, therefore, is based on six major constructs (see Figure 10.3), with a central focus on strategic management. The complementary constructs are community, transformational leadership, harmony, transitions, and the learning organization.

Community is an aggregate of individuals and teams who create a common vision and values, and interact to create structures and systems to achieve their shared goals. Members share a sense of belonging and commitment to the organization's goals and objectives. A community is a composite of its past, present, and future. Learning opportunities are provided for new and continuing members. Community members participate in decision making and problem solving about interdependent activities, space, and resources (Bellah et al., 1985; Friedman, 1993; Gardner, 1991).

Transformational leadership is an orientation to facilitating change in groups and/or organizations. The mission of the transformational leader is to engage individuals and groups in shifting to new mental models or paradigms of how to relate to each other to accomplish common goals. Transformational leadership is based on the deliberate use of values and principles to empower people (Covey, 1991). In this new perspective on leadership, the would-be leader is characterized by a guiding vision, passion, integrity, trust, curiosity, and daring. In addition, Bennis outlined four traits of leadership: attention, meaning, trust, and self (Bennis, 1986). In the CDM, the transformational leader values sound management and provides resources and guidance to achieve common goals.

The *Harmony Principle* is a fitting, orderly, and pleasant joining of diversities (Boje, 1991; Doczi, 1985). Creating harmony requires attention to social, psychological, and physical environments. A formula has been proposed by Boje for designing organizational change that results in a good fit between people and their environment (Rhythm plus Contrast with Emphasis in Balance equals Harmony). The formula has five related principles: Plan for rhythm that gives pace to the work; promote variety in unity; build in contrast; design changes with emphasis on the organizational vision; and work to achieve balance.

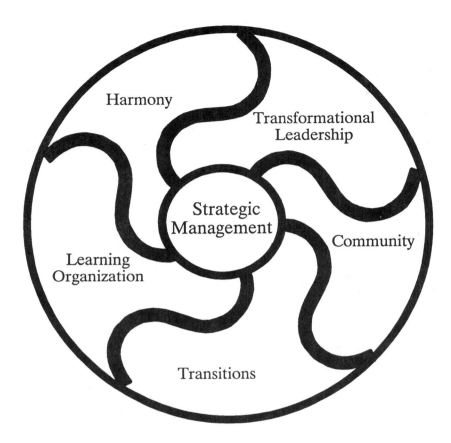

Figure 10.3. Community Design Model Conceptual Framework

Transitions are an internal process precipitated by change that people and organizations go through to come to terms with their new situation (Bridges, 1991). There are three stages of transition: the *ending* (the way we were in the past), the *neutral zone* (the set of conditions and activities that must take place to move from the present to the future), and the *beginning* (the way we will be in the future). Major groups of transitions are triggered by a variety of changes: developmental, maturational (puberty, pregnancy, retirement); situational (death of a relative, job layoffs); health/illness (acute and chronic changes); and organizational shifts. At a time of transition, there is an openness and vulnerability to interventions that support the individual or group through the process of adjustment.

A *learning organization* is an organization that discovers how to tap into people's commitment and capacity to learn, at *all* levels in the organization. There are five disciplines in a learning organization (Senge, 1990, p. 4): systems thinking, personal mastery, mental models, building a shared vision, and team learning.

These conceptual framework constructs drive the development of strategic direction structures and systems tailored to the setting, reflect the desired culture, determine necessary competencies, and provide direction for measurement of outcome indicators (Jewell & Jewell, 1992).

Strategic directions are a means of operationalizing the vision or moving from "vapor to paper and paper to practice" (J. Miura, personal communication, March 1992). The assumption in the CDM is that attention to the following four strategic directions will create an organization that is long-lasting and responsive to changes that support quality, customer-centered outcomes, quality work life, and organizational effectiveness.

In the CDM, strategic management comprises visioning and valuing, planning, implementation, monitoring, and evaluation. An essential element of strategic management in this model is an orientation to "interactive, backwards planning" described by Ackoff (most recently in a conversation reported in the Healthcare Forum, Flower, 1992). Key elements are designing the future you want (as opposed to guessing what might happen) and working "backwards" from your vision of where you want to be to the current reality. Ackoff proposes that this planning approach that transforms the sense of what is possible requires systems thinking (Ackoff, cited in Flower, 1992; Senge, 1990). The assumption is that what is really important about a system is its essence as a whole. According to Ackoff, "A system is a consequence of the way its parts interact, not the way they act" (cited in Flower, 1992, p. 64). Systems operate through interactions, and, to be effective, organizations need to manage these interactions. This is in contrast to former management strategies of taking a system apart, managing activities, and solving problems in isolation.

The strategic directions of the CDM are creation of a community initiative, establishment of a leadership culture of continuous improvement, development of a user-friendly environment that empowers stakeholders, and development of systems to facilitate transitions.

Community initiative is an organizational spirit or effort to act from shared vision and values that emphasizes the development of a sense of community in all aspects of organizational life, independent of geography, department, and discipline. All stakeholders are members of the community.

Leadership culture of continuous improvement is a commitment to instilling a conviction that every stakeholder is a leader who is accountable for creating and using opportunities for improvement that contribute to achieving shared outcomes.

A *user-friendly environment* is a climate in which harmony is created by empowering individuals and groups to create customer-centered systems that balance diversity and alignment.

Transition systems are mechanisms to assist individuals, groups, and the organization to cope with changes by providing time and space, resources, coaching, and anticipatory guidance.

The strategic directions in an organizational design model are a template for implementing the activities that will accomplish the goals. Flexibility in interpretation of these directions is essential in the meaningful application across settings.

Indicators

In this model, the assumption is that quality patient care, a quality work life, and organizational effectiveness will be the primary outcomes. Outcomes are achieved by implementing the strategic directions. For each strategic direction, indicators will be found in the following areas: culture, structures, systems, and learning/competencies. These indicators were adapted from the 7-S framework described by Peters and Waterman (Waterman, 1987).

Culture is the vision, the values, the goals, and what a group stands for as reflected in how things are done. Culture simplifies everyday life by providing rules and expectations for interacting with others (Thiederman, 1991). Within an organization, values influence the prevailing paradigms that shape practices and in turn create norms for appropriate behavior. Cultural values are demonstrated not only in interactions but in the symbolic behavior and style of the organization (for example, observe the art on the walls, ways memos and other communications are delivered, dress, and celebrations).

Structure defines and demonstrates the integration of the roles and relationships of people in the company and the functional relationships of equipment, people, and facilities. Structures are designed to focus on teamwork, empowerment, a sense of belonging, decentralized decision making, and the development of human potential. The structures required to support the reengineering need to address developing interdependence through teams, shared decision making at the service level, and communication and governance across the institution.

Organization-wide restructuring encompasses both the strategic management process and the cultural process. *Strategic process* relates to what needs to be done. This process includes the broad strategic goals to be achieved in support of the mission and vision, the specific objectives set to accomplish those goals, and the tasks that must be performed to meet specified objectives.

A *system* is a network of interdependent relationships and processes in a complex dynamic balance. Systems shape how things get done day to day. Organizations and service units are interrelated sets of systems. Communication, decision making, and work take place within boundaries and follow patterns. Actions in one part of the system have consequences for other parts of the system that create tension/stress. Goals are achieved by balancing feedback and flexibility through formal and informal mechanisms (Senge, 1990; User Friendly Environment Strategic Direction Council, 1993; Waterman, 1987).

Learning is the acquisition of skills and understandings. Reflection-in-action (Schön, 1990) becomes a primary framework for learning. *Competence* is the application of those skills and understandings to accomplish goals and the work to be done. Organizing around core competencies allows for flexibility in responding to external shifts and pressures (Wheatley, 1992). The strategic plan derived from the CDM will address building a profile of competencies rather than a profile of service units.

Processes

The CDM outlines various processes that support restructuring through reengineering. Processes for facilitating change are critical to successful implementation of the model. These are the use of interactive planning in strategic management, attention to transition management, values and vision, flattened hierarchies, recognition and rewards, information flow, and development of a learning organization. The methods to accomplish this are work redesign, role reconceptualization, systems development, leadership development, and team building. We will highlight two processes central to application of the CDM in any setting. These are strategic management and transition management.

Creating constellations that illustrate the interrelationships and linkages among the plan elements (strategies) is a critical step for involving broad groups of stakeholders in the restructuring process (Nazarey, 1993). As a framework for thinking about strategies, constellations identify all aspects of the strategy and serve as a blueprint for action planning. Analysis of this type helps to reveal linkages between strategic plan elements, as well as providing the opportunity for organizational connectivity. Developing constellations helps to identify resource needs. Constellations are developed at the organization level by a team of executives and key formal leaders in the organization. Drafts of constellations are taken to staff at the service level for refinement and linkages. Constellations have the four elements and indicators that describe outcomes.

Service-level people begin action planning with an environmental scan for strengths, weaknesses, opportunities, and threats. They operate on four themes of reengineering: process orientation, rule breaking, ambition, and creative use of information technology (Hammer & Champy, 1993). Action planning aims at work designs that "neither compromise the integrity of people to achieve work efficiency nor compromise productivity to make people happy" (Hackman, 1980, cited in Tonges, 1992, p. 27).

Successful work redesign occurs when work units change from functional departments to process teams; jobs change from simple tasks to multidimensional work; people's roles change from controlled to empowered; and job preparation changes from training to education. "The approach is aimed at creating work situations in which teams instead of individuals have a whole and meaningful part" (Lawler, 1992, p. 88). Evaluation is designed around the four indicators: culture, systems, structures, and learning/competence.

To implement the CDM, a *transition management* structure is established. As we shift from a system perspective that focuses on interactions among people, processes, and design (rather than problem solving), transitions become more critical. Change is accomplished by shaping teams that cross traditional boundaries and levels. The pattern of representation in the structure is designed to create a microcosm of the key stakeholders in the organization. The structure makes provisions for continuous involvement of top executives who empower stakeholders. Ultimately, the organization must integrate the transition management structure into a permanent structure, using the CDM components to oversee strategic management over time.

MODEL APPLICATION: WORK IN PROGRESS

We will begin the description of our application with a historical perspective. Progress will be addressed in terms of the four CDM outcome indicators: culture, structures, systems, and learning/competence. Changes at the organizational (reengineering) and service (work redesign) levels will be highlighted.

The CDM was initiated by the nursing executive team in collaboration with key stakeholder groups at Harbor-UCLA Medical Center. The Strengthening Hospital Nursing Program, funded by the Robert Wood Johnson Foundation/Pew Charitable Trusts, was the impetus for integrating Nursing Department innovations under way in the medical center to achieve a unified, interdisciplinary model for change.

Harbor-UCLA Medical Center is a university-affiliated hospital in an urban area of southern California. The medical center serves over 2 million residents of southwestern Los Angeles County, predominantly young and culturally diverse. The center is spread out over 72 acres and combines a 553-bed tertiary care hospital, over 100 ambulatory care clinics, the Research and Education Institute, Inc., a faculty private practice, and cooperative ventures for research and innovative services. More than half of the patient population is Hispanic, 16% is white, and 15% is black (Harbor-UCLA Medical Center, 1992).

The goal of the CDM is to realize the vision of becoming a "Community of Patient Care Leaders" (CPCL), in which everyone is a leader and a member of our campus community. In this vision, primary care would become the basis of interaction with patients and "WE CARE" the acronym for our shared values. (Vision and values statements available from the authors.)[1]

In 1989, a small team in the Department of Nursing at Harbor-UCLA Medical Center prepared a planning grant to facilitate broad-scale organizational change. A Design Team was created consisting of the Directors of Nursing, Medicine, and Hospital Administration as well as the division directors for Professional Practice Affairs and for Research in the Department of Nursing and the associate hospital administrator for Operations. From this team, a vision for the medical center restructuring emerged that emphasized reengineering using our theoretical constructs, with special emphasis on creating an internal sense of community and recognition of each individual stakeholder as a leader.

Tentative strategic directions were drafted, and four planning teams were commissioned to begin the strategic planning process. Working from the vision and their sense of current reality, the teams used an interactive, backwards planning approach. Each team compiled assessment data and generated recommendations that were the foundation for the CDM and a Harbor-UCLA strategic plan.

A transition management framework for the CDM was developed. an Executive Steering Council (ESC) and four Strategic Direction Councils (SDCs) were established (specifics to be detailed later). The primary mission of both the ESC and SDCs is to implement the strategic plan for restructuring to a CPCL. On the basis of this vision, the strategic plan outlines activities that are organized under the four indicators of the CDM (culture, structures, systems, and learning/competence). We will briefly describe below the major activities and lessons learned through model application.

Culture

Restructuring to a CPCL creates new expectations for behaviors and invites individuals to reexamine their core values and beliefs. The major shift is for previously fragmented and insulated groups and departments to come together across boundaries as a community. The CDM conceptual framework and the CPCL vision and values provide the base for these cultural shifts. Specific changes include enculturating the following values: leadership and continuous quality improvement, teams, cultural/diversity sensitivity, harmony, and the learning organization.

Cultural processes relate to how things should be done: key values implied by the agreed-on mission and vision, specific group practices to support the values, and behaviors of individuals representing those values. Aligning these two aspects of restructuring—implementing the strategic plan and making the necessary cultural changes to support restructuring activities—is a continuing challenge. Harbor-UCLA has been a predominantly experiential, task, and data-driven organization. We are transitioning to a new model of leadership in which individuals and teams are more autonomous, participatory, and involved in the decisions that affect their work life, patient care, and the effectiveness of the organization.

Restructuring to a CPCL challenges us to become deliberate, plan oriented, and values driven. It has therefore been extremely useful to highlight and maintain a balance between strategy implementation and cultural change, as well as to demonstrate early results and successes of pilot projects.

Developing a shared language is a critical vehicle for cultural change. The challenge is to maintain a balance between new terminology (and the crucial messages it carries) and comfort levels. Communications to various stakeholders should be sensitive to cultural diversity, experience with the restructuring efforts, and organizational level and style. It is important to build upon what people are most accustomed to and to make strong connections between the new and the familiar.

Cultural change needs to be modeled from the top of the organization. At Harbor-UCLA a shift has begun from executive Design Team leadership to decentralized, multileveled decision making and strategic management. This mind-set has led to a flattened hierarchy within transition management groups. The esprit de corps observed within the executive team created a renewed interest in involvement from other stakeholders. Enrolling others in the vision has been essential to broadening the leadership base.

All teams related to the CPCL have staff as members. Everyone has a voice and contributes to results. These include not only staff nurses but clerks and other assistants. Considerable energy was required initially to coach and reassure these individuals that they were to participate as equal members. For example, when a vote was called, they often required specific invitations to voice their decision.

Small group meetings become a primary arena to accomplish the broad-scale change prescribed by the organization's application of the CDM. In our experience, meetings are often a microcosm of the organization. Agendas and interactions reflect the status of the change efforts. Decision making takes on new importance as a tool for empowerment. Capitalizing on this, our meetings are constructed to model appropriate behaviors that reflect our vision and planned cultural changes. Neutral, third-party facilitators help to ensure that goals are met, and conversations are constructed with special attention to listening and reflection, issues of diversity, and win/win agreements (Covey, 1991; Leonard, 1991). The facilitator acts as the chauffeur so that the group coleaders can participate in the group process.

Strategic management moves the reengineeering vision from planning to implementation. Implementation begins at the organizational level with creating a plan with strategic directions.

Structures

Structures were planned to bring the CDM application to the service level. These include minicommunities, community councils, and leadership teams. At Harbor-UCLA, the early minicommunities included Ambulatory Care (Cardiology) and Perinatal. Various community councils have emerged as a prelude to minicommunity development in the Emergency Department for Adult Care, Pediatrics, and Obstetrics/Gynecology. Leadership Teams emerged around pain management (both adult and pediatric), skin care, tuberculosis, reimbursement, staff recognition, and the shift to managed care.

The minicommunity development is an example of work redesign at the service level. The primary goal is to provide quality, patient-centered care, with careful attention to a quality work life and organizational effectiveness. Minicommunities are new ways to support collaboration among key groups who relate to the patient and the family. In order to focus on results, work units change from functional departments to process teams. The assumption is that it is easier to make changes in the environment than to reshape behavior. Each team is empowered to make decisions about its work and assume responsibility for the outcomes. Different disciplines who formerly worked in a parallel play or in isolation are now integrated across disciplines and geographical boundaries in patient-centered process teams. The role of the formal leader is to provide vision and to coach and inspire others to develop their leadership potential (Marriner-Tomey, 1993). For some health care providers, this expectation that everyone is a leader is a major paradigm shift, especially when it encompasses the patient and family.

Additional structural components evolved, such as external partnerships with the larger community: for example, the University of California at Los Angeles School of Nursing faculty, the *Los Angeles Times,* and the Center for Case Management. Partnerships with on-campus groups such as the local chapter of the National Management Association and the Research and Education Institute also emerged. Projected structures include development of models for leadership and a user-friendly environment, patient and staff resource centers and a leadership center to support leadership development and transitions, an Office of Community Affairs, an Environment Board, and a new organizational governance structure.

The transition management structure at Harbor-UCLA Medical Center consists of four interrelated groups. The Design Team, which sets the direction for restructuring, functions in an advisory capacity to the other groups. The Design Team provides leadership with respect to vision and strategic directions and is responsible for making resources available. Members of this group include representatives from the executive leadership ranks of the organization.

The Design Team is also a subset of the larger group known as the Executive Steering Council (ESC). The primary focus of this council is to plan, lead, and facilitate the management and implementation of restructuring and to communicate the restructuring throughout the organization. This group has 36 members representative of major role groups on campus. A primary role for the ESC is to charter, coordinate, and give direction to four Strategic Direction Councils. These councils correspond to each of the four strategic areas of restructuring: creation of a community initiative, establishment of a leadership culture of continuous improvement, development of a user-friendly environment that empowers stakeholders, and development of systems to facilitate transitions. The mission of each council is to oversee and make implementation decisions as each strategic direction is brought to life.

The reengineering of the organization level moves to the service/customer level through Process Action Teams (PATs). At Harbor-UCLA, each council identifies and charters PATs that will implement strategic restructuring activities (Process Action Team, undated). It is the council that asks why we do what we do. When that becomes clear, processes are identified that will facilitate the organizational reengineering. Process is a collection of activities that takes one or more types of input and creates an output that is of value to the customer.

The PATs, with members who are close to the process, undertake necessary work redesign. They achieve agreement on the council's vision of the ideal process, conduct analyses of the current situation, and create innovative programs, systems, and structures that support their new view of the process. The PATs monitor the results of implementing their changes and assist the council in evaluating the effectiveness of the new process in light of the overall organizational strategic plan.

In addition, through this transition, formal and informal links were drawn to existing medical center structures, such as the Administrative Council and standing committees. In some instances, this created a parallel structure that would have to become integrated over time.

Systems

The focus is on developing systems to support cross-campus communication, access to information, and integration among all systems. Specific activities include the development of systems thinking throughout the organization, a campus-wide systems improvement plan, a stakeholder-centered communication plan, stakeholder participation systems, reward and recognition systems, indexes for transitions, transition management skills and awareness, and a Patient Care Atlas map series (to include role, critical path, geography, and team responsibility maps).

Implicit in all systems is work redesign at the service level. Work redesign guidelines (Hammer, 1990) are illustrated with examples that emerged in our setting:

1. *Put the decision at the point where the work is performed and build control into the process.* In the past, the nurse manager and physician would have decided what should happen to patients in a certain diagnostic group. With work redesign, the entire team (those who are closest to the point of service)—staff nurses, aides, and clerks—collaborated with the nurse manager, physician, clinical nurse specialist, midwives, social workers and nurse practitioners to develop a critical path.

2. *Organize around outcomes not tasks.* Quality care is assessed not by whether all the perinatal patients got Sitz baths, but by whether readmissions and emergency room visits decreased.

3. *Have those who use the output of the process perform the process.* In the past, patients' diets were adjusted based on lab values obtained many hours after the specimen. Now, using automated technology, nurses collect the specimens and analyze the results immediately.

4. *Subsume information processing work into the real work that produces the information.* Instead of sending data on critical path variance to the quality improvement coordinator, the staff track and analyze their own data and initiate changes as needed.

5. *Treat geographically dispersed resources as though they were centralized.* Members of the team may have home departments (and offices) away from the clinical unit. In a minicommunity, they share a common responsibility for patient care outcomes. This sharing is reflected in granting access to home base resources, personal case notes, computer databases, and equipment, and building in time for reflection and team development activities.

6. *Link parallel activities instead of integrating their results.* The traditional pattern of interdisciplinary, provider-driven parallel play is disrupted, and all members of the team coordinate their work around the patient's experience. This means that team membership is not optional (Lawler, 1992). To increase the sense of shared responsibility as well as to accomplish a number of other objectives, members of the work team are typically cross-trained so they can do most, if not all, of the tasks that fall within their work team's area of responsibility. According to Lawler, members usually rotate among tasks on a regular basis. This type of training not only gives the work group flexibility in assigning members but also gives people a sense of ownership and responsibility for the final product.

7. *Capture information once and at the source.* Documentation was time consuming and frustrating in its redundancy. Nursing notes were eliminated and a multidisciplinary record instituted to minimize time spent reconciling discrepancies. The hospital information system is being customized to support efficient data sharing across the interdisciplinary team.

Learning/Competence

Restructuring to a CPCL invites individuals and groups to redefine the work to be done and reexamine their core values and beliefs. In many cases, new skills and/or knowledge require intensive training and reorientation. Core competencies include leadership, patient-focused care, systems thinking, transition management, role theory, team building, cultural/diversity sensitivity, and community-building initiatives.

We have learned to give particular attention to building community through the ways we interact with each other. Small-group settings provide the opportunity to explore techniques such as dialogue and reflection, civility, willingness to take risks (individually and collectively), and appreciation of diversity in backgrounds, personalities, questions posed, learning styles, frames of inquiry, and spectrums of interpretation (Christensen, 1991).

Where concepts and techniques are more innovative and outside of the scope of what is traditionally taught in nursing and medical schools, the training needs are particularly demanding. We have offered some specialized instruction and facilitation training both on and off campus while building a train-the-trainer program.

The challenge for managers and staff is in learning to let go and give guidelines, work within those guidelines, delegate while still remaining in the loop, and encourage autonomy and accountability without creating chaos. In the process of moving decisions closer to the work, it has become apparent that all stakeholders need to understand and use clear decision-making guidelines. The format we found helpful was to appreciate that the leader needed to determine whether buy-in or time was the major factor. For example, when the guideline is that the leader will "decide and announce," the time required is minimal, but so is buy-in. The subsequent levels require increasing time but build great ownership. These levels include gathering input from individuals, gathering input from the group, determining consensus from the group, and delegating the decision to a subgroup (Interaction Associates, 1987).

Evaluation

For each of the strategic directions, evaluation encompasses the four indicators (culture, structures, systems, and learning). In order to assess the reengineering and related work redesign, a variety of methodologies are being used. For example, cultural changes are assessed with standardized questionnaires, interviews and unobtrusive measures (Webb, Campbell, Schwartz, & Sechrist, 1966). Systems are evaluated as an organic whole (Wheatley, 1992), with attention to patterns that engage both people and the environment. Specific focus is on eliminating rework and duplication, minimizing variance, and maximizing resources. Structures are examined in terms of their efficiency and harmony with the environment. Learning/competence is measured in terms of both process and outcomes. The achievement of specific competencies is linked to the extent of application in multiple settings. Attention is paid to dissemination beyond the original learners. In addition, the learning activities are evaluated for their effectiveness in creating the anticipated outcomes. In all cases, both qualitative and quantitative methods are used.

CONCLUSIONS

> To get people to move from where they are to where they are supposed to be requires two actions. First, they have to get unstuck from where they are. The tool that unsticks people is a wedge—the case for action. Next, the unstuck people have to be attracted to another point of view. That is the job of a magnet—the vision. (Hammer & Champy, 1993, p. 155)

Reengineering provides the leverage through which broad-scale organizational change becomes a reality. The CDM, coupled with an organization's vision, provides the design to create and strategically manage the future.

NOTE

1. Paula Siler, RN, MS, Harbor-UCLA Medical Center, 1000 West Carson, Box 482, Torrance, CA 90509. Phone: (310) 222-3409.

REFERENCES

Bellah, R., Madsen, R., Sullivan, W., Sidler, A., & Tipton, S. (1985). *Habits of the heart*. Berkeley: University of California Press.

Bennis, W. G. (1986). Four traits of leadership. In J. Williamson (Ed.), *The leader-manager* (pp. 79-89). New York, NY: John Wiley.

Bennis, W. G. (1989). *On becoming a leader.* Reading, MA: Addison-Wesley.

Boje, D. M. (1991, March). *The classical principles of organization design.* Unpublished paper, Loyola Marymount University, College of Business Administration, Los Angeles.

Bridges, W. (1991). *Managing transitions: Making the most of change.* Reading, MA: Addison-Wesley.

Christensen, C. R. (1991). Premises and practices of discussion teaching. In C. R. Christensen, D. A. Garvin, & A. Sweet (Eds.), *Education for judgment: The artistry of discussion leadership* (pp. 15-34). Boston: Harvard Business School Press.

Covey, S. R. (1991). *Principle-centered leadership.* New York: Summit.

Department of Nursing. (1990, May). *Harbor-UCLA Medical Center: A community of patient care leaders transitioning to a culture of empowerment* [grant proposal]. Torrance, CA: Harbor-UCLA Research and Education Institute, Inc.

Doczi, G. (1985). *The power of limits: Proportional harmonies in nature, art and architecture.* Boston: Shambala.

Etzioni, A. (1993). *The spirit of community: Rights, responsibilities, and the communitarian agenda.* New York: Crown.

Flower, J. (1992, March/April). New tools, new thinking. *Healthcare Forum Journal,* pp. 62-67.

Friedman, E. (1993, May/June). Concepts of community. *Healthcare Forum Journal,* pp. 11-17.

Gardner, J. W. (1991). *Building community.* Washington, DC: Independent Sector.

Hammer, M. (1990, July-August). Reengineering work: Don't automate, obliterate (pp. 104-112).

Hammer, M., & Champy, J. (1993). *Reengineering the corporation: A manifesto for business revolution.* New York: Harper Collins.

Harbor-UCLA Medical Center. (1992). *Hospital profile: Fiscal year 1991-92.* Torrance, CA: Author.

Helgesen, S. (1990). *The female advantage: Women's ways of leadership.* New York: Doubleday.

Imai, M. (1986). *Kaizen: The key to Japanese success.* New York: Random House.

Interaction Associates. (1987). *The complete facilitator* [learning program]. San Francisco: Author.

Jewell, S. F., & Jewell, D. O. (1992). Organization design. In H. D. Stolovitch & E. J. Keeps (Eds.), *Handbook of human performance technology: A comprehensive guide for analyzing and solving performance problems in organizations* (pp. 211-232). San Francisco: Jossey-Bass.

Lawler, E. E. (1992). *The ultimate advantage: Creating the high-involvement organization* (pp. 77-121). San Francisco: Jossey-Bass.

Leonard, H. B. (1991). With open ears: Listening and the art of discussion leading. In C. R. Christensen, D. A. Garvin, & A. Sweet (Eds.), *Education for judgment: The artistry of discussion leadership* (pp. 137-151). Boston: Harvard Business School Press.

Liu, M., Denis, H., Kolodny, H., & Stymne, B. (1990). Organization design for technological change. *Human Relations, 43*(1), 7-22.

Marriner-Tomey, A. (1993). *Transformational leadership in nursing.* St. Louis, MO: Mosby Year Book.

Milgrom, P. R. (1988). Employment contracts, influence activities, and efficient organization design. *Journal of Political Economy, 96*(11), 42-59.

Nazarey, P. J. (1993, April). *From vapor to paper: Restructuring to a community of patient care leaders.* Paper presented at the American Organization of Nurse Executives Annual Meeting, Orlando, FL.

Process Action Team. (undated). *Treatment of sexually transmitted diseases* [Process Action Team story]. San Diego: San Diego Naval Hospital.

Senge, P. M. (1990). *The fifth discipline: The art and practice of the learning organization.* New York: Doubleday.

Schön, D. A. (1990). *Educating the reflective practitioner.* San Francisco: Jossey-Bass.

Thiederman, S. (1991). *Bridging cultural barriers for corporate success: How to manage the multicultural work force.* Lexington, MA: Lexington.

Tonges, M. C. (1992, January). Work designs: Sociotechnical systems for patient care delivery. *Nursing Management,* pp. 27-32.

User Friendly Environment Strategic Direction Council. (1993). *Proceedings.* Torrance, CA: Harbor-UCLA Medical Center.

Waterman, R. H. (1987). *The renewal factor: How the best get and keep the competitive edge.* New York: Bantam.

Webb, E., Campbell, D. T., Schwartz, R. D., & Sechrist, L. (1966). *Unobtrusive measures: Nonreactive research in the social sciences.* Chicago: Rand McNally.

Wheatley, M. J. (1992). *Leadership and the new science: Learning about organization from an orderly universe.* San Francisco: Berrett-Koehler.

CHAPTER 11

Restructuring a Nursing Organization: A Vision to Meet 21st-Century Challenges

Nashat Zuraikat
Patricia Hillebrand
Andrea Catania Cocovich
Teri Ficcichy
Cynthia Shirley

This chapter describes the experience of a 176-bed acute care facility serving a rural population of 45,000 in western Pennsylvania, in utilizing a job design strategy to reorganize the nursing structure, establish a clinical ladder, and increase the nurses' satisfaction in decision making. In 1989, a 5-year plan was developed to decentralize the decision-making process and establish a unit-based nursing delivery system that included unit managers, patient care specialists, and continuous quality coordinators. The title of head nurse was changed to unit manager. The initial phase of the plan was conducted over 2 years to train the unit managers in management and financial skills. At the same time the management training was being done, the central nursing office continued to provide some centralized functions like staffing, scheduling, and quality assurance. New unit manager functions were phased in over the 2-year training period. The number of unit managers was reduced from eight to six, and the positions of patient care specialist and continuous quality coordinator were created. The patient care specialist's function was to assist the unit manager in facilitating the process of patient care. In addition, the patient care specialist was responsible for coaching the staff nurse in collaborative practice with physicians and other department managers and also for patient advocacy and family liaison. The continuous quality coordinator was responsible for quality reviews for assuring competency in the skill labs, preceptor training, and criteria of the Joint Commission on Accreditation of Healthcare Organizations (JCAHO). The members of the management team collaborate on each nursing unit to provide a unified delivery system.

The challenges facing nursing executives in the United States today are staggering. With the pressure to continue the provision of quality patient care on one hand and to continue to cut costs on the other, the nurse executive finds the necessity of maintaining a healthy balance one of the most fundamental challenges. Health care expenditures continue to rise faster than the inflation rate. Health care spending reached $808 billion in 1992, almost 13% of the Gross Domestic Product. This compared to $250 billion or 8.3% in 1980. Spending is projected to reach $1.7 trillion or 20% of the GDP by 2000. The United States spends more per capita on health care than any other country on the face of the earth ("Health Care Reform Cost," 1993). The workload of nursing continues to grow in complexity due to radical changes in expanding technology (Baillie, Trygstad, & Cordoni, 1989). In addition, the tension resulting from comparative shopping by the consumer is escalating, and the pressure of managed competition is on the horizon. With the impact of all these challenges occurring on nursing units, one way the system can be managed for quality and cost-effectiveness is to decentralize and redesign the nursing organization to provide unit-based management. Redesign of nursing organizations has been suggested as a way to reduce cost and increase productivity and work commitment to meet the challenge of the future (McDaniel & Stumpf, 1993; Stewart, 1992).

This chapter will review the experience of one facility in the utilization of job redesign strategies to reorganize the nursing management structure, to establish a format for clinical ladders, to increase the nurses' job satisfaction, and to promote quality patient care while reducing the cost of hospital care. The development and implementation of the nursing restructure process are also discussed.

THE DEVELOPMENT OF THE REDESIGN

Historical Overview

Prior to 1990 restructuring, the nursing management team consisted of nursing directors, head nurses (unit managers), assistant unit managers, shift coordinators, a staffing coordinator, and a quality assurance coordinator (see

TABLE 11.1 Comparison of Nursing Positions

Before Reorganization	After Reorganization
9 unit managers	6 unit managers
8 assistant unit managers	10 patient care specialists
4.5 shift coordinators (supervisors)	3 shift coordinators (supervisors)
1 GRASP coordinator	4.5 continuous quality coordinators
1 quality assurance coordinator	1 risk management specialist
1 clinical orientation coordinator	
24.5 total FTEs	24.5 total FTEs

Table 11.1). The nursing department was hierarchical in structure and central-ized in function (see Figure 11.1).

In 1989, a 5-year strategic nursing plan was developed. The goal of the plan was to develop strategies that would revitalize the nursing department. The an-ticipated outcomes were more efficiency in the delivery of patient care, more effectiveness in the use of managerial skills, increased staff satisfaction, and improved recruitment and retention. Because the nursing department was cen-tralized at that time, the plan to become a decentralized unit-based manage-ment system needed to be developed and phased in over a 5-year period. The plan outlined the vision; however, the organizational culture was not ready to make the transition. Therefore, a number of strategies designed to promote personal and managerial growth were developed. Initially, the objectives fo-cused on the development of a multilevel communication and education system within the Nursing Department that included a biweekly newsletter, monthly staff luncheons, and retention committees on each unit. Expansion of educational opportunities to include offering of prepaid tuition reimburse-ment to encourage staff at all levels to return to school and the offering of increased inservice and staff development activities were initiated. In addition, the existing head nurse title was changed to unit manager, and monthly managerial education programs for the nurse managers were provided. Ac-cording to del Bueno (1991), the purposes of restructuring the work of head nurses or unit managers are to provide greater job satisfaction, improve out-comes for patients, nurses and the organization, and empower the professional nurse's role.

PHYSICAL ENVIRONMENT

The strategic plan also addressed the issue of space. The nursing philosophy for each unit was spelled out. The nurses were asked to do pilot projects on the

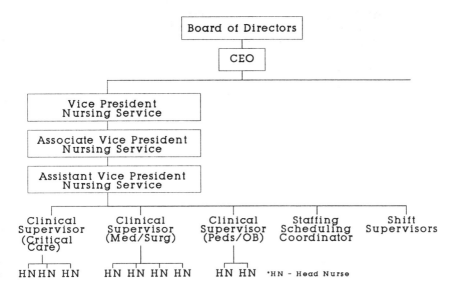

Figure 11.1. Hierarchical/Centralized Structure of Nursing Department Before Restructuring

units to define how functions should be carried out. The process they used was similar to what Davidhizar (1992) called *nemawashi*. *Nemawashi* is the process by which an unofficial understanding is reached before an official decision is made to encourage creativity and innovation by nursing staff. The pilot projects led to the redesign of the nursing unit to provide the staff nurse with the most efficient work space possible. The pilot projects also provided the front-line staff with the opportunity to experiment with change in a nonthreatening way. The existing 46-bed nursing units were each divided into two smaller units of 23 beds. Nursing stations were located closer to the patients, and patient servers (compartments for storage of medication, equipment, and supplies) were added. Patients were clustered according to specific needs.

BUILDING TRUST RELATIONSHIPS

According to Jenkins (1992), adequate time and effort in training and education are major components to ensure effective and successful work redesign. The long-term goal of the plan was to build a trust relationship over time that would create a climate in which the front-line patient care providers would experience more autonomy and would be more ready to participate in the development of clinical ladders. Once again, strategies were developed to assist the staff in the transition. This was necessary because the process of change may be traumatic and thus resistance to change may occur even when the need for change is recognized (Harter, Grossman, Swank, & Spring, 1989). One of the strategies was to ask the staff which job-related factors were most important to them. Because change may be threatening, information relating to the need for change, plans for change, and consequences of change must be shared with the staff. The staff were encouraged to conduct and participate in research to find out what factors were most important to them in their jobs. Over a 1-year period, three research projects were conducted in the hospital. One study showed that the nurses were least satisfied with the hospital's administrative policies and with advancement and recognition opportunities (Hung, 1991). The second study revealed that the majority of nurses were dissatisfied with centralized decision making and communication (Zuraikat, 1990). The third study revealed that scheduling was a major dissatisfaction variable (Shirley, 1991). In addition, the data revealed that nurses were dissatisfied with their ability to be involved in decision making. The nurses felt they received no positive feedback or recognition, and had little ability to control their work environment. The results of the research provided valuable information to move the restructuring forward. The nursing units were given guidelines to assist them with scheduling, and each unit began to self-schedule. In addition, nursing staff from every unit were regularly invited to lunch with the vice president for Patient Services, and weekly rounds by nursing administrators were begun on all shifts. The goals were to enhance communication between the staff and nursing administration and to reduce the staff's anxiety.

Throughout the initial phase of the plan, while the head nurses were being educated in the management skills necessary to manage their units, the central nursing office continued to provide some centralized functions, namely, quality assurance and staffing/scheduling based on a patient acuity system.

Over the next 2 years, the training program continued to enhance leadership and management skills of the unit managers. All nurse managers attended monthly classes on the principles of management, and the components of the 24-hour unit manager's position were delegated and performed by them, step by step.

TRANSITION

Initially, nurse managers in the new positions struggled with the responsibilities of their new role. They repeatedly expressed deep conflict between the desire to do hands-on clinical work and the desire to perform the new duties assigned, which included independent decision making.

The unit managers slowly started to understand and accept the scope and responsibility of their new role. However, conflicts started to emerge between some unit managers and the staff carrying out the centralized functions in the nursing office. All of the players experienced a great deal of role confusion.

In addition to the interpersonal conflict and confusion, some of the missing resource allocation issues began to emerge. The following issues were identified:

1. Each year there were a number of new graduate nurses hired, and the unit manager had no time in her new role to ensure that those new nurses were well prepared for their practice.
2. The requirements of the total quality improvement system were overwhelming.
3. The unit managers could not keep pace with the day-to-day management of the unit, plus meet all these additional challenges.
4. Under the previous, centralized management system, the head nurse had been the primary communicator on patient care issues with physicians and other providers of care. As the nurse manager's role changed, the need to educate the front-line nurses on collaborative practice skills became apparent.

RESTRUCTURING

The restructuring of the nursing department consisted of two phases. The first phase was moving from a centralized to a decentralized structure. The second phase was job redesign to clearly delineate the roles of all the essential components of the system.

In January 1992, the next step in the development of the new structure was initiated. All the nurse managers were asked to provide suggestions on what each felt were essential components for the nursing department. All the information submitted was used to design the new structure (Figure 11.2). The managers were also asked to identify problems encountered in Phase 1 of the restructuring.

PROBLEMS IDENTIFIED

The following problems were identified on the basis of the unit managers' feedback and what is reported in the literature:

1. The unit manager needed resources at the unit level to ensure that nursing process and patient teaching were occurring.
2. Resources were required to provide unit-based quality improvement by analysis of quality issues. This included providing education and training when problems were identified.

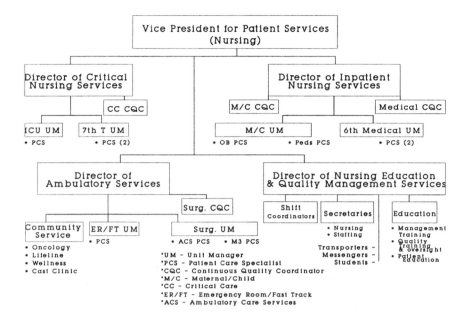

Figure 11.2. Structure of Nursing Department During the Transition

3. The increased age of our patients pointed to a need to assure patients and families that a patient advocate would be available to discuss their concerns.
4. There was a need for a unit educator to provide skill labs to ensure the competency of all caregivers on a continual basis.
5. There was a need for resources to ensure that all units' policies and procedures were reviewed regularly and that the staff was kept informed of current policy.
6. Staff knowledge of JCAHO criteria, quality improvement necessity, and patient acuity system designation was essential.
7. The unit managers needed more time to ensure that the business elements of their position were addressed.

In addition, the positions of the American Nurses Association (1988), American Hospital Association (1992), and JCAHO (1992) on the role and function of the hospital nurse manager were reviewed. From the information available, several issues were identified:

1. The Nursing Department's vision and values needed to be congruent with those of the hospital.
2. The nurse managers of the future would need to be prepared at least at the baccalaureate level.

3. The nurse managers would need to be at department manager level within the organization.

ESSENTIAL COMPONENTS

The Nursing Department's strategic vision must be congruent with the hospital's vision. To ensure that nursing's vision and values were consistent with those of the hospital, the vice president for Patient Services developed a workshop to enable the administrative staff, department managers, unit managers, and first-line supervisors to explore their visions for the hospital. Over a 3-month period of time, management groups worked to define their vision for the hospital for the year 2000. Once each group had captured its vision, it worked to define the values and culture necessary to accomplish that vision. The result of this work was the basis for the hospital's strategic plan. The nurse managers were also asked to define the essential components of the nursing structure in conjunction with the development of the hospital's strategic plan.

Because of the hospital's financial situation, it was clear that no new full-time-equivalent (FTE) positions could be added to the new structure. Only currently allocated positions were utilized.

Job descriptions were developed outlining the specific needs identified. Units were clustered and consolidated, and the number of unit managers was dropped from nine to six. The day shift coordinator (supervisor) position was eliminated, reducing FTEs from 4.5 to 3. The acuity system coordinator and the quality assurance coordinator positions were abolished. The assistant unit manager position was changed to a patient care specialist position, and the number of these positions was increased from 8 to 10 (no more than 24 patients per patient care specialist). The position of continuous quality coordinator was created, and 4.5 FTEs were allocated to this position. A risk management specialist position was created that had hospital-wide responsibilities. The key duties of each of these positions are outlined in Table 11.2. The goals of the restructuring are outlined in Table 11.3.

Because a goal of the nursing plan was to empower the front-line nurses and give them autonomy, it was essential to provide consistent coaching on all shifts. Educational requirements were established for each job classification, and those selected were required to enroll in the appropriate educational program within 6 months of assuming the new position.

All 25 nurses currently involved in management were invited to apply for the available positions. They were interviewed by the nursing directors and the vice president for Patient Services. The final candidates for unit manager were

TABLE 11.2 Essential Elements of Each Position

Unit Manager (N = 6)
- Recruits and selects personnel
- Evaluates performance/discipline
- Formulates and monitors budgets
- Responsible for compliance with all state, JCAHO, and regulatory agencies
- Supervises staffing/scheduling
- Accountable for nursing care given
- Maintains harmonious relationships between assigned unit, medical staff, other departments
- Analyzes systems and problem-solves for efficiency
- Focus on customer relations

Shift Coordinator (N = 3)
- Functions as an extension of administration and is responsible for coordinating the activities of all hospital departments during their shift
- Supervises and coordinates activities of nursing personnel on an 8-hour tour of duty when unit managers are not present.
- Participates in interpretation of policies of Indiana Hospital and the nursing department to all hospital employees and physicians
- Contributes to budget planning, control, and evaluation
- Provides supervision for staff and initiates corrective action in conjunction with unit managers
- Does staffing adjustments
- Reviews assignment sheets on nursing units
- Investigates complaints and begins problem-solving strategies
- Coordinates admissions

Patient Care Specialist (N = 10) (1/24 ratio)
- Ensures that nursing process is implemented on all patients
- Ensures that all pertinent information is recorded and legible
- Makes regular patient rounds independent of physician
- Coaches nursing staff on physician/nurse communication process
- Assigns staff and makes staffing adjustments
- Resolves conflict
- Focus on customer satisfaction—actively listens for feedback
- Coordinates patient movement for studies and transfers
- Works collaboratively across department lines to ensure that focus remains on what is best for the patient (patient advocate)

Continuous Quality Coordinator (N = 4.5)
- Conducts educational programs for assigned areas in the following subjects: CQI, GRASP, JCAHO, Skill Labs
- Unit resources persons for CQI: leads quality circles, develops indicators, assists staff with analysis of data, oversees report submission
- Unit resource person for GRASP: reviews and revises GRASP charts, orients new staff to GRASP system, active member of GRASP committees
- Conducts training of staff on regulatory review requirements
- Ensures all policy manuals are current and staff informed of any updates
- Coordinates the orientation, teaching, and continuing development of staff, including preceptor training and development of a consistent preceptor training schedule
- Reviews incident reports and routes—provides training to assess reduction of occurrences

TABLE 11.3 The Goals of the Restructuring

To realign resources to provide the best possible patient care and maintain a liaison among patients, their physicians, health care providers, and the patient's family

To focus on empowerment of nurses by continuing the process of decentralization identified in the Nursing 5-Year Plan

To cluster like units to free the maximum number of nurses for patient care and liaison duties

To increase the number of patient care specialists to facilitate the process of patient care

To move support resources to the unit level to ensure staff knowledge and competency are maintained in the areas of patient care, total quality management, and the acuity system

To prepare the department for the implementation of career/clinical ladders within nursing as defined in the 5-Year Plan

To provide a system of consistent preceptor training to ensure that all new employees receive a comprehensive orientation program, and to ensure that ongoing technical skill training is provided to maintain and document staff competency

To focus patient advocate services on the nursing units to assure that they are available for patients and families as needed

To provide nursing staff with coaching for collaborative practice skills to ensure that the patient's needs are addressed by the physicians and other hospital departments

To continue to develop customer awareness and the necessity of dealing with patients, families, physicians, and internal departments from a customer service philosophy

To build an alliance with the institution of higher education in nursing so that collaboration and dialogue can occur

also interviewed by the vice president for Human Resources, vice president for Medical Affairs, and the president and CEO.

Prior to the completion of the interviews, the staff involved were experiencing increased stress. The Hospital's Employee Assistance Program (EAP) provider met with them to provide stress reduction strategies and assistance in coping with change. Once the selection process was completed, an intensive education and training program was initiated.

EDUCATION

In preparation for changes that would occur with the restructuring of the Nursing Department, a plan was developed that simultaneously addressed the emotional needs of all those affected by the changes and focused on accomplishing the goals established.

Lewin's (1951) theory of change and the processes involved in change was used as the basis for planning an educational program. Consideration was given to identifying all those who would be affected by the change, what effects the change would have (Welch, 1990), and obstacles, such as employee resistance to change, that could potentially occur (New & Couillard, 1990).

The overall educational strategy included using open and direct two-way communication regarding changes throughout the execution of each phase of the restructuring. The purpose of this was to lay the foundation for the development of teamwork and trust through active staff participation. Ritter and Tongas (1991) noted this factor as essential for successful implementation of new delivery systems for patient care.

Initially, meetings were held to inform all levels of nursing staff, physicians, faculties of affiliating schools of nursing, hospital board members, non-nursing department managers, and administrative staff of the purpose and goals of the restructuring. Question and answer periods were allotted at each session in an attempt to dispel any personal fears or concerns that arose due to the restructuring. Topics addressed included concern over change in employment status, change in job responsibilities at the staff nurse level, and concern that restructuring would cause decreased staffing. In addition, an open-door policy for answering questions at times other than scheduled meetings was adopted by the Vice President for Patient Services, nursing directors, shift coordinators, and unit managers. This policy was communicated to all persons involved in the change process.

The educational plan then focused on meeting the needs of the nurse managers directly affected by role change. To assist the nurse managers in adapting to and succeeding in their new role requirements, a management course was developed. The course included ways to find solutions to the problems identified in the previous structure of the nursing department and methods to use to fulfill goals established. Malcolm Knowles' theory on how adults learn served as a reference point for designing the management course (Kidd, 1973, pp. 36-38; Knowles, 1970).

Knowles' concept of *andragogy,* the art and science of leading adult learning, proposes that adults are self-directed, have an orientation to learning that is problem centered, and have a need for immediacy of application. The climate for learning for the adult must be one in which there is respectful collaboration, and should not be authority oriented (Knowles, 1973).

Mindful of these concepts, the management course included a variety of teaching techniques to hold the managers' interests and provided the managers with an opportunity to use their self-directedness through the use of role play. The course was presented over a 4-month period and began before the official starting date of the restructuring to provide the nurse managers with an ongoing forum for discussing their own anxieties about the change. Classes were held separately for unit managers and shift coordinators, patient care specialists, and continuous quality coordinators in order to provide an opportunity to concentrate on the specific needs of each group.

The first session included a review of the job description pertinent to each group, and defined role perceptions and expectations. The remainder of the course included subject matter familiar to all managers. However, to be meaningful, the course included practical application methods to use in the nurse manager's particular setting. Assignments required that group members provide examples of how they had used material discussed in class in the actual clinical setting with their staff members. A critique was then done on their actions to reinforce their learning and application and to change behavior if needed.

In keeping with Knowles' concept that adult learning occurs if subject matter is timely, the course content for all groups included topics that would have immediate application in the nurse managers' interactions with staff. These topics included review of leadership styles, use of positive management to achieve desired results, group process and team building, theory of change and resistance to change, the importance of self-empowerment and empowerment of staff members, effective communication, assertiveness techniques, time management and delegation, problem solving and decision making, and goal development. The role of the manager relative to regulatory agency requirements, quality management, and the patient acuity system was also defined and explored.

Additional teaching/learning sessions were held to discuss topics that were specific for each group.

IMPLEMENTATION

Once the design of the system and the position selection process were completed, implementation was started. New roles were unofficially assumed 6 weeks prior to the official start date. The 6-week period was provided to reduce anxiety in all those involved. During this time, meetings were held every

2 weeks with the entire group to review problems identified and to ensure operational consistency across all units. At the end of the 6-week period, roles were assumed officially. The unit managers and shift coordinators were given department manager status. All 24 involved were placed on 6 months' probation, with monthly appraisal designed to provide them feedback on their progress. At the end of the 6-month probationary period, two of the nursing director positions were abolished. The two employees involved were transferred to the Hospital Planning Department, where additional resources were needed.

The transition began in 1990 and was completed in 1993. The total nurse manager positions in 1990 included the 24 involved in the reorganization plus three clinical supervisors, an associate vice president, and an assistant vice president. The total positions in July 1993, at the end of the transition, included the 24 positions and two nursing directors. Four high-level nursing administrative positions were eliminated. In addition, the Vice President for Nursing position was changed to a Vice President for Patient Services, and additional hospital departments were added to her area of administrative responsibility. Figure 11.3 shows the final structure.

Because one of the dissatisfaction factors among the nurses was an inability to control their work environment, a strategy for clinical/career ladder development was initiated (see Figure 11.4). According to Sovie,

> Hospitals able to design and implement a successful nursing practice career plan will be the magnet hospitals of the future. They will become institutions where professional nurses are recognized and valued for their contributions to patient care, where professional nursing is practiced, and finally, where nurses advance in career patterns that are personally and professionally satisfying. (Sovie, 1982, p. 6)

The development of the clinical/career ladder criteria is currently in process. The structure has been finalized, and staff committees are being formed to start the process of defining the specific requirements for each level. The number of clinical specialists will be limited to one per specialty. Their role will be one of consultant to the nurses within that specialty.

PROMOTION

Because one of the goals of the nursing plan was to assist with the recruitment and retention of nurses, a promotion strategy was developed.

As part of a promotional effort to communicate the nursing department's redesign, a poster presentation was done at an affiliated university's graduate

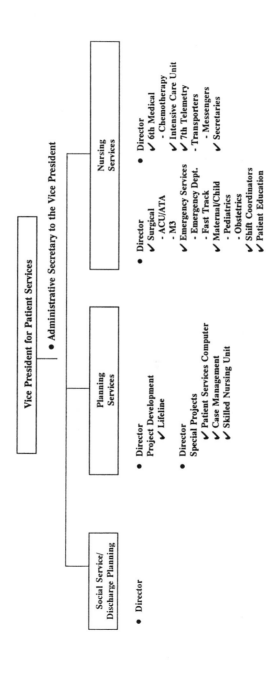

Figure 11.3. Structure of Nursing Department at the Completion of the Project

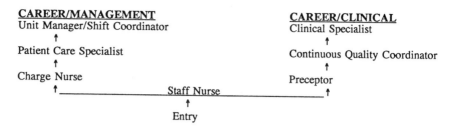

CAREER/MANAGEMENT   **CAREER/CLINICAL**
Unit Manager/Shift Coordinator   Clinical Specialist
↑   ↑
Patient Care Specialist   Continuous Quality Coordinator
↑   ↑
Charge Nurse   Preceptor
↑_____ Staff Nurse _____↑
↑
Entry

Figure 11.4. Career/Clinical Ladder Model

nursing program. The poster session presented a graphic display of the patient-centered model and described the institutional position supported by the reorganization. The poster emphasized the specific changes in responsibilities of the unit managers, patient care specialists, continuous quality coordinators, and shift coordinators. The goals of the new structure were well outlined and presented in an easy-to-read format. The focus of the nursing redesign is the patient, and the nursing organization is built outward from the patient. The poster session clearly demonstrated the shift from a centralized to a decentralized structure.

One of the purposes in presenting the poster session at the university was to further enhance the bonds between the hospital and the university. The quality of the hospital staff and the facility is important in building the hospital's image in the community. Through communication, strong bonds and affiliations with the local university help ensure that the organization's redesign is understood.

Communicating the organization's beliefs is an ongoing process and should include all those involved with the organization. The university's presence in the hospital is an important component of providing quality care in the community. Further collaboration between the institutions will improve care as well as ensure that mutual goals are attained.

CONCLUSIONS

The vision for our hospital for the year 2000 is that it will be a delivery system in which patient care is the main emphasis. That system will be built on teamwork and trust, with continuous quality improvement activity across departmental lines guiding the hospital forward. According to Hinshaw, Smeltzer, and Atwood (1987), an environment in which nurses can grow and thrive professionally will positively affect the quality of patient care. The nursing department believes that the redesign will contribute to the success of the hospital in reaching that vision.

Hospitals will increasingly rely on the labor of nonphysicians (such as registered nurses and physician's assistants) to provide low-cost health care. In 1989, when the strategic plan was developed, the threats that would overshadow the health care environment in 1993 and beyond could not have been predicted. However, the plan has provided a road map of planned change that is assisting the organization in continuing to move forward in turbulent times. The hidden benefit has been the initiation of an environment in which change is viewed as the norm and employees are empowered to actively participate as designers and engineers of the change process (Tornabeni & DeBaca, 1991).

The future of the health care delivery system is in question. Hospitals will face a drastic reduction in reimbursement that will require a complete redesign of the way they function ("Health Care Reform Cost," 1993). The redesign of the nursing structure in this hospital has provided a basic framework within which all levels of staff can function. The hierarchical structure has been flattened, and the resources have been shifted to the nursing units, thus reducing cost. The unit management structure is designed to provide coaching for the front-line staff on collaborative, problem-solving skills. It is hoped that this work will reflect positively on patient satisfaction, quality of care, and nurses' job satisfaction. As additional changes affect the health care delivery system, the model and the framework will provide the stability needed for the staff to meet future challenges.

REFERENCES

American Hospital Association. (1992). *Role and function of the hospital nurse.* Chicago: Author.

American Nurses Association. (1988). *Standards for organized nursing services.* Kansas City: Author.

Baillie, V. K., Trygstad, L., & Cordoni, T. I. (1989). *Effective nursing leadership: A practical guide.* Rockville, MD: Aspen.

Davidhizar, R. (1992, August). What nurse managers can learn from Japanese management style. *Today's O.R. Nurse, 14,* 33-37.

del Bueno, D. (1991). Managers: Frustration and form in the new organization. *Journal of Nursing Administration, 5*(21), 46.

Harter, C., Grossman, L., Swank, E., & Spring, B. (1989). Networking to implement effective health care. *American Journal of Maternal Child Nursing, 14*(6), 387, 390, 392.

Health care reform cost. (1993). *Pulse: The Health Care Reform Newsletter, 1*(1), 12-16.

Hinshaw, A., Smeltzer, C., & Atwood, J. (1987). Innovative retention strategies for nursing staff. *Journal of Nursing Administration, 17*(6), 8-16.

Hung, L. (1991). *Staff nurses' job satisfaction.* Unpublished manuscript.

Jenkins, J. (1992). Work redesign: Ensuring services. *Aspen's Advisor for Nurse Executives, 7*(10), 4-6.

Joint Commission on Accreditation of Healthcare Organizations (JCAHO). (1992). *Accreditation manual for hospitals: 1992—Nursing care standard 5.* Oakbrook Terrace, IL: Author.

Kidd, J. (1973). *How adults learn.* Chicago: Follett.

Knowles, M. (1970). *The modern practice of education.* New York: Association Press.

Knowles, M. (1973). *The adult learner: A neglected species.* Houston, TX: Gulf.

Lewin, K. (1951). *Field theory in social sciences.* New York: Harper & Row.

McDaniel, C., & Stumpf, L. (1993). The organizational culture: Implications for nursing service. *Journal of Nursing Administration, 23*(4), 54-60.

New, J., & Couillard, N. (1990). Guidelines for introducing change. In E. Hein & M. Nicholson (Eds.), *Contemporary leadership behavior: Selected readings* (3rd ed., pp. 311-317). Glenview, IL: Scott Foresman.

Ritter, J., & Tongas, M. (1991). Work redesign in high intensity environments. *Journal of Nursing Administration, 12*(21), 26-35.

Shirley, C. B. (1991). *Job satisfaction related to self scheduling and ill time.* Unpublished manuscript.

Sovie, M. (1982). Fostering professional nursing careers in hospitals: the role of staff development, part I. *Journal of Nursing Administration, 12*(12) 5-10.

Stewart, A. C. (1992). Redesigning the system: Radical work redesign is needed to truly focus on patient needs. *Journal of Neuroscience Nursing, 24*(4), 179-180.

Tornabeni, J., & DeBaca, V. (1991). Restructuring, redesign: Laying the groundwork. *Aspen's Advisor for Nurse Executives, 7*(2), 8.

Welch, L. (1990). Planned change in nursing. In E. Hein & M. Nicholson (Eds.), *Contemporary leadership behavior: Selected readings* (3rd ed., pp. 299-309). Glenview, IL: Scott Foresman.

Zuraikat, N. (1990). *Determinants of intention to leave among Indiana hospital registered nurses.* Unpublished manuscript.

ADDITIONAL READINGS

Bocchino, C. (1991). An interview with Steven A. Shroeder, president of the Robert Wood Johnson Foundation. *Nursing Economics, 9*(6), 383-390, 400.

DeBock, V., & Waite, R. (1988). Consumer response: A reflection on change. National Commission on Nursing Implementation Project to restructure nursing practice. *Nursing Administration Quarterly, 12*(3), 57-59.

Mercy Health Services: Systemwide redesign of patient care services. (1991). *Nursing Administration Quarterly, 16*(1), 38-45.

O'Malley, J. (1991). The redesign agenda: Changes in service delivery. *Aspen's Advisor for Nurse Executives, 6*(11), 2.

Roch, R. (1992). Overview of health care restructuring within current resources. *Canadian Journal of Nursing Administration, 5*(2), 8-11.

Vosburgh, N. (1991). Product line management through organizational redesign. *Nursing Administration Quarterly, 15*(2), 39-45.

CHAPTER 12

Patient-Centered Differentiation: Laying the Groundwork for an Interdisciplinary Model for Care Delivery

Cheryl B. Stetler
Nancy Sheets

This chapter will address the complex issue of differentiation of nursing practice in the context of a restructuring project at Hartford Hospital. It will provide a brief description of this newly evolved Patient-Centered Redesign Program, including expectations regarding differentiation. The latter is defined as distinguishing levels of practice and related competencies, activities, and expectations among various roles within a professional department or across departments, where applicable. It will then present an innovative model for differentiated staffing that takes this concept beyond nursing and provides a vehicle for unfreezing old paradigms and operationalizing new concepts of patient-centeredness, collaboration, and cost efficiency. Informa-

AUTHORS' NOTE: Acknowledgment is given to the jointly sponsored grant from the Robert Wood Johnson Foundation and the Pew Charitable Trusts, "Strengthening Hospital Nursing: A Program to Improve Patient Care," and to the National Program Office. Their support helped to make this innovation in differentiation possible. The valuable contribution of many individuals made this chapter possible. Although the individual names of so many fine clinicians cannot be listed, the work of the subgroup that helped to develop the initial differentiated staffing model is noteworthy: Beth Greig, Pat Montanaro, Dr. Pat Maher, Shirley Wightman, and Mary Canning.

tion on use of the model, resultant perceptions of nurse managers and others involved in the process, and factors that facilitate and hinder its application will be described.

Differentiation, no matter how it is defined, is a difficult concept to operationalize (Goertzen, 1991). If based on educational preparation, as in Primm's approach (1987), it can evoke strong emotional reactions and thus resistance. In addition, such educational requirements may be difficult to fully enact where there is a scarcity of baccalaureate graduates.

If differentiation is based on competency and experience, it can still fall short of its expectations: For example, clinical ladders designed to differentiate practice can instead reward longevity or other attributes unrelated to patient care outcomes, and attempts to modify assignment expectations according to patient needs can evoke resistance because of perceived inequities in resultant workloads. This resistance unfortunately can be related to the perception that "indirect work" such as care planning or coordination is not "equal" to physical/technical work (i.e., equally heavy or equally useful). It can also be related to the fact that clinical ladder differentiation often focused on nurses' needs (to grow, develop, advance, or receive increased remuneration; see Murray, 1993) rather than on a set of patient needs that identify requirements for a specific mix of staff.

In any differentiation scenario, the issue of understanding the difference between "mutual valuing of roles versus equality of roles" is sure to be encountered (Milton, Verran, Murdaugh, & Gerber, 1991, p. 285). So too is the need to identify a creative, useful methodology by which a conceptual differentiation framework can be converted into an operational staffing mix.

Introduction of differentiation is obviously a major challenge to the status quo of any nursing department. It requires not only commitment, but also innovative methods to facilitate effective implementation. Furthermore, it has implications for choice of a practice model. This includes definition of the basic nature of nursing as well as the role of nonlicensed support staff and interdisciplinary collaboration. McClure (1991, p. 5) suggests that "a practice model can only succeed if it uses patient needs as its basis and is congruent with the role[s] and functions that fulfill those needs" (plural of "role" added). In today's health care environment, there is growing recognition that collaboration and interdisciplinary teamwork are essential if organizations are to survive and thrive (National Program Office, 1992). Such collaboration requires appreciation not only that different roles fulfill different functions, but also that a key driving force in that determination is patient needs. This fact, in addition to an increasing need for cost efficiencies in resource utilization, leads to a realization that differentiation is no longer solely a nursing issue.

This chapter describes the initial experiences of Hartford Hospital with differentiation and a related model for differentiated staffing. The context of organizational restructuring, entitled the Patient-Centered Redesign Program (PCR), will first be provided, including the related role of differentiation. This will be followed by a brief introduction to a conceptual differentiation framework. The remainder of the chapter will present the differentiated staffing model in detail, including examples of the latter's use within nursing and with interdisciplinary groups. Issues, barriers, and progress reported by individuals who participated in this creative approach to change will be presented.

PATIENT-CENTERED REDESIGN PROGRAM

In 1990, Hartford Hospital became one of 12 hospitals and eight consortia nationwide chosen to receive $1 million under the jointly sponsored grant from the Robert Wood Johnson Foundation and the Pew Charitable Trusts, "Strengthening Hospital Nursing: A Program to Improve Patient Care" (National Program Office, 1992). The title of Hartford's project became known as Patient-Centered Redesign, and had as its vision the "creation of an innovative, patient-centered, hospitalwide delivery system that continuously improves quality and utilizes resources cost effectively" (Hartford Hospital, 1990). From its inception, Hartford's Program focused on the overall delivery system rather than nursing per se, and was expected to involve all departments and disciplines. Its widely disseminated objectives and core principles continually reinforced this fact throughout the organization (see Table 12.1), and over time, interdisciplinary and interdepartmental collaboration became a pervasive, integrating theme for almost all activity at the clinical and managerial level.

Despite this critical organizational focus, specific aspects of nursing were to be implicitly or explicitly transformed. These reflected back to barriers to practice identified in the initial "request for proposal":

- Lack of differentiation of levels of practice among registered nurses and its relationship to a model for scope of practice and nursing care delivery
- Lack of clear delineation of authority, accountability, and coordination relative to direct patient care activity among all health care workers, as well as the related definition of nursing versus non-nursing tasks
- Hospital systems that were not designed to optimally support the delivery of cost-effective patient care

TABLE 12.1 Overview of Hartford Hospital's Patient-Centered Redesign Program

Core Principles[a]

1. *Patient-Centeredness:* Everything done at Hartford Hospital is recognized as a patient-related event; *patients* are the reason we are ALL at the hospital.

2. *Collaboration:* In order to meet the needs of our patients, we must first work together as a team; only *together* can we continuously improve what is in essence an integrated system.

3. *Participation: Everyone* must be involved in redesign and implementation of this integrated delivery system; this means relentlessly wanting to continuously improve everything we do for whomever we do it.

4. *Outcomes:* We must all focus on the *results* of our collective efforts, in relation to both the cost of our delivery system and to patient outcomes.

Objectives of the Program

1. *Redesign of organizational systems* at the tactical (nursing unit), operational (service/department), and strategic (hospital-wide) levels to improve productivity, utilize resources cost-effectively, and enhance systemwide quality/outcomes achievement

2. *Redesign of collaborative practice* to integrate functions of nurses, physicians, and other professionals

3. *Redesign of information systems* to affirm advances in technology, monitor productivity, and provide necessary information for patient outcomes assessment and decision making

SOURCE: a. Taken from an internal communication.

Out of these barriers and objectives, primarily redesign of collaborative practice, came a set of innovations or changes that were to be introduced through Patient-Centered Redesign:

1. Differentiation of nursing practice, in which the belief that "a nurse is not a nurse" was to be operationalized through daily competency-based assignments and routines.

2. Within this differentiation model, creation of a patient care coordinator (PCC) role somewhat similar to that of a case manager. The PCC role was to be an integral part of nursing differentiation and episode-related, interdisciplinary Health Care Teams.

3. Development of innovative, alternative multiskilled employee (MSE) roles. These roles were to enable provision of cost-effective delivery of care to a specific patient population and, in addition, to relieve nursing of non-nursing tasks. This innovation was thus also related to differentiation.

4. Unit-based redesign, in which patient-related innovations would come together in a new, idealized delivery system at the unit and service level: for example, differentiation, MSEs, Health Care Teams, and PCCs, as well as targeted system and managerial changes and the use of clinical paths.

Need for Nursing Differentiation

On the basis of the success of a collaborative practice pilot project, primary nursing was accepted in the 1980s as the Hartford Hospital Department of Nursing's model for practice (Koerner & Armstrong, 1983). Also in the 1980s a clinical ladder system was introduced, primarily as a tool for recruitment and retention. Its focus was on recognition of a nurse's accomplishments or potential for growth.

The extent to which primary nursing "took" throughout Hartford Hospital varied. On some units, it was implemented in a manner consistent with the conceptual intent and philosophy of the model. On other units, primary nursing was accepted as a modality but not operationalized in a manner consistent with its basic philosophy and intent. Sample factors that influenced this state of affairs, and that can be found in like institutions, include the following: new, creative scheduling patterns that were convenient for staff but militated against the concept of continuity; assignment of "primary nursing responsibilities" to nurses without sufficient competencies to fulfill its expectations; lack of understanding of the essence of "operationalizing" key concepts of the primary nursing model (e.g., 24-hour accountability); and basic barriers to practice that resulted in a poor use of professional nursing time (e.g., time spent cleaning sitz baths or filling in for other professionals not available on off-shifts).

As for the clinical ladder system, it afforded an opportunity for growth, development, and increased remuneration as a nurse progressed through three steps. In day-to-day activities of a unit, however, the most expert nurses were often given the same type of assignment as novice or "competent" nurses. On some units, staff wanted the workload of RNs (of any level) and LPNs or Patient Care Assistants to be "equal." That meant "fairly and evenly" dividing the patients among all "caregivers." In reality, the underlying assumption that Clinical III nurses had more expertise than Clinical I nurses was not always translated into a differential use of their talents. Clinical IIIs were more likely to be given the "resource" or charge nurse assignment, but their clinical talents and time, within an optimal cost-benefit ratio, given the salary of such expert nurses, were not put to the best use. Given this situation, the hospital's nursing leadership felt that the Strengthening Hospital Nursing Grant was a prime opportunity and time to truly differentiate nursing practice.

Competency-Based Nursing Differentiation

Differentiation, within Patient-Centered Redesign, was defined as distinguishing levels of practice and related competencies, activities, and expectations among and within various roles. It applied to individual professional roles, specifically the registered nurse, and could be utilized both within single departments and across departments, where applicable.

The overall purpose of differentiation was to (a) facilitate the most appropriate and cost-effective use of each member of a unit/department, in order to provide the best possible outcomes for patients; (b) make explicit the importance, value, and discriminating (i.e., differentiating) characteristics of more complex professional activities, such as coordination; and (c) operationalize, in daily assignments, progressive levels of critical thinking among different registered nurses. Within nursing, the eventual subgoals of differentiation focused on operationalization of critical aspects of practice, such as:

- Making daily assignments that appropriately match the needs of patients with nurses' and assistant personnel's competencies
- Developing an appropriate staffing mix and scheduling pattern that match the needs of patients with nurses' and assistant personnel's competencies
- Clearly defining an individual nurse's level of accountability and supporting that specific level of practice

Differentiation and the related concept of behaviorally defined competency were to be central components in the review and revision of nursing practice at Hartford Hospital. They would be key concepts in development of an overall nursing model (see Kron & Gray, 1987) and in the evolution of Patient-Centered Redesign. The approach taken, however, had to be consistent with the overall culture of Hartford Hospital (see Armstrong & Stetler, 1991). Given this organizational culture, it was presumed that a strict educational approach to change (e.g., Primm, 1987; Wolahan, 1991) was not viable.

Only the Department of Nursing was initially involved in focusing on differentiation and the related redesign of a professional practice model. The steps that were initially undertaken in this process included the following:

1. *Clarification of values and assumptions for nursing practice* (see Table 12.2 for beliefs about differentiation). Patient-centered care, holistic nursing care, competency-based nursing practice, coordination, the nursing process, and collaboration were core concepts that emerged.

2. *Outline of a values-based conceptual framework for differentiation of nursing practice.* This began to define levels of practice. Higher levels were defined as those requiring more critical thinking and more comprehensive accountability. Neither educational nor orientation needs of new graduates or other staff were included.

TABLE 12.2 Core Values Regarding Differentiation of Nursing Practice

---

Although all staff will be responsible for practicing in accordance with professional standards, their position, level, sophistication of application, and compensation will be differentiated according to the following:

  a. level of competency
  b. education
  c. experience
  d. preference

Appropriate, advanced nursing education will prepare a nurse for a more advanced level on the continuum of practice. This continuum of competency can be expressed through progressive stages of development, ending with advanced practice. Differentiation of nursing practice will, therefore, identify multiple responsibilities and varying degrees of complexity along this continuum. This will be done in relationship to

  a. predictability of patient care needs
  b. level of complexity of patient care needs
  c. discrimination of specific actions that will provide
     the best possible outcomes for patients and families

"Professional" behaviors such as committee participation and continuing education, though important, were also not considered as part of the differentiation of practice.

3. *Development of measurable, behavioral details regarding patient-focused levels of practice.*

Working from the foundation of the above values and framework, an Ad Hoc Differentiation Group began to develop behavioral details regarding differentiation across levels. For example, the predictability and complexity of patient needs in relation to practice behaviors were routinely considered across the nonlicensed, multiskilled employee; LPN; competent RN; proficient RN; expert RN; and advanced RN/PCC levels.

A review of the literature was conducted but did not provide models with the practice detail or focus desired. However, the American Nurses Association Social Policy Statement (1980), literature on case management, and some of Benner's (1984) novice-expert concepts were influential factors.

After many months of work, a Differentiation Competency Document that outlines explicit and progressive practice behaviors was developed (separate manuscript under preparation). Assessment, Planning, Intervention, Outcome Evaluation, and Coordination were used as organizing categories. Each category in turn was broken down into relevant subcategories of practice, for example, within Assessment, data collection, interpretation, and problem identification.

A DIFFERENTIATED STAFFING MODEL

Once a conceptual framework and a tool to assess the level of individual staff competency were available, the next major task was twofold: (a) to find a strategy to help head nurses and relevant others convert this view of competencies into a new, understandable paradigm of practice and (b) to identify a methodology that would help operationalize it within the day-to-day staffing and delivery system. It was also important that these activities converge with other components of the Patient-Centered Redesign Program to create unit-based redesign. This phase would integrate differentiation with the concepts of multiskilled employees, health care teams, clinical paths, and an episode of care focus. A "Differentiated Staffing Model" (DSM) was identified as a possible means of achieving the above.

The DSM model is a step-by-step process designed to assist key staff in rethinking, reframing, and redesigning the type of staff—nurses and other caregivers, both licensed and nonlicensed—needed to meet a population of patients' needs. It is based on the assumption, a là Ackoff (1981), that a visionary unit cannot be created by focusing on what happens now; rather, redesign must start with (a) what patients need and (b) an idealized view of what care should be, rather than what it currently is. This includes eliminating what does not need to be done. It also includes creatively envisioning how care can be delivered in a totally different manner. In the end, the DSM process is designed to facilitate identification of

- The levels of nurses required to meet the needs of a specific group of patients (e.g., LPNs and/or competent RNs, and/or proficient RNs)
- Multiple, need-related activities that could collectively be used to more clearly define new multiskilled employee roles
- Nonnursing professionals who are needed to meet specific unit-based patient needs and their ability to do so, given current practice systems
- Given the above, the interdisciplinary staff mix or proportion of each identified category and level that would be needed on a redesigned unit

The steps used in this expert, judgment-based process are briefly described below. Tables 12.3 through 12.5 present related visual tools and instructions used in differentiated staffing sessions. Table 12.6 provides a sample from one

TABLE 12.3 Focus of Patient Needs Identification

Categories of Patient Needs	Description
Health restoration	Patient needs related to the reason for hospitalization that are be-ing intervened on by the health care team to facilitate the patient's return to his/her optimal level of functioning/wellness prior to current episode: i.e., treatment needs (medical, nursing, and allied health); and preventive needs relative to potential of disease/treat-ment-related complications
Health maintenance	Patient daily functional needs/patterns that are being maintained by the health care team at his/her baseline level during current episode: e.g., mobility, hygiene, fluids, nutrition, comfort, pre-vention of complications related to being hospitalized/bedridden, such as injury, immobility, constipation, bedsores
Health promotion	Critical patient needs that are being intervened on by the health care team through patient/family involvement to promote recov-ery and an optimal postdischarge level of health relative to reason for hospitalization and other critical needs as appropriate: i.e., teaching and discharge planning for self-care needs; encouraging patient to the optimal level of independence (medical, nursing, and allied health); preventative maintenance such as immuniza-tions; vision, hearing, and dental testing; pap smears, cholesterol levels
Environmental	Patient needs for comfort/safety that are met via use of unit-based resources such as equipment and supplies: i.e., provision of light-ing, furniture, supplies, TV, meals, water, amenities, linens, pre-admission set-ups, unit-based equipment
Coordination systems	Patient needs that are met via diverse hospital-based systems (i.e., communication, collaboration, transport, maintenance of unit-based equipment, access to equipment) and community-wide systems (i.e., referrals to VNA, social services, long-term care facil-ities, protective services, etc.)

such session. Before their explication, several influential factors and learnings should be noted.

First, during initial efforts to identify the need for and potential types of new, multiskilled employee roles, no concrete method was available to keep the assigned work groups focused on a futuristic viewpoint. Participants had difficulty staying focused on what patients needed, what should ideally be done, and who ideally should do it. Rather, they kept reverting to information that was currently available in terms of traditional roles and traditional time/motion-management engineering methods. Data were therefore generated that "rearranged the deck chairs" but did not fulfill the differentiation or overall

(text continued on page 179)

TABLE 12.4 Differentiation of Staffing Model—Phase I

Focus: A comprehensive view/verification of a group of patients' needs from the perspective of the health care team.[a]

Patient Needs Categories[b]	Total %	High	Med	Low	Components of Care (Assess, Plan, Intervene, Evaluate, Coordinate)
Health restoration[b]					
Health maintenance					
Health promotion					
Environmental					
Coordination systems					
Total	100%				

Steps:

1. Identify the major population groups for your unit (maximum number = _____); choose one to begin the differentiation process.

2. Determine the nature of the patient needs in this population within each category (health restoration, etc.); assess in terms of typical activities or elements of care. Assign the proportionate percentage of overall needs to each individual category under the "Total %" column. The total must equal 100%.

3. Identify and discuss the complexity of the identified needs in each category; assess in terms of typical activities or elements of care and level of expertise required of health care team to meet that need.

4. Subdivide the allocation for each major category across the three levels of complexity until all boxes are filled (0% is an option). Vertical and horizontal percentages must sum appropriately. Example: If 30% of the group's needs fall into the category of health restoration, determine what portion of these needs are of high, medium, and/or low complexity, such as 20%, 5% and 5%, respectively.

5. (Optional; after Phase II) Estimate relative time requirements of activities per level of complexity. Do this by subdividing the percentage figure allocated to each category as follows: e.g., if 30% of patients' overall needs relate to health restoration, then decide how that figure of 30% should be subdivided across high-, medium-, and low-complexity activities to illustrate the proportionate workload related to each level.

a. Health care team—a multidisciplinary group of health care providers that intervene to meet the needs of a specific patient population.

b. See Table 12.3 for definitions of categories of patient needs.

TABLE 12.5 Differentiation of Staffing Model—Phase II

Focus: Identification of each discipline/role's contribution to meet the patient needs identified in Phase I (High-Complexity Calculation Page)

Patient Needs Categories	Total %	DISCIPLINE							
Health restoration		HIGH-COMPLEXITY TOTAL ___ (Total % from Phase I ___)							
Health maintenance		HIGH-COMPLEXITY TOTAL ___ (Total % from Phase I ___)							
Health promotion		HIGH-COMPLEXITY TOTAL ___ (Total % from Phase I ___)							
Environmental		HIGH-COMPLEXITY TOTAL ___ (Total % from Phase I ___)							
Coordination Systems		HIGH-COMPLEXITY TOTAL ___ (Total % from Phase I ___)							

Steps:

1. Identify and list the disciplines/roles involved or potentially involved in the care of the population under analysis.

2. Transfer the high-complexity totals determined in Phase I to their respective categories.

3. Determine the most cost-effective disciplines/roles that can meet the various activities in this category, given this level of complexity. Subdivide the total accordingly; every discipline/role may not contribute to every need or level of expertise.

4. Total the columns vertically for each discipline/role to obtain each's total contribution for the high-complexity level. Complete the medium- and low-complexity pages, and then obtain a grand total per discipline/role.

177

TABLE 12.6 Sample Completed Form From a Differentiated Staffing Session

Focus: A comprehensive view/verification of a group of patients' needs from the perspective of the health care team.[a]

Patient Needs Categories[b]	Total %	Components of Care (Assess, Plan, Intervene, Evaluate, Coordinate)		
		High	Med	Low
Health restoration[b]	30			
Health maintenance	20			
Health promotion	30			
Environmental	10			
Coordination systems	10			
Total	100%			

Steps:

1. Identify the major population groups for your unit (maximum number = _____); choose one to begin the differentiation process.
2. Determine the nature of the patient needs in this population within each category (health restoration, etc.); assess in terms of typical activities or elements of care. Assign the proportionate percentage of overall needs to each individual category under the "Total %" column. The total must equal 100%.
3. Identify and discuss the complexity of the identified needs in each category; assess in terms of typical activities or elements of care and level of expertise required of health care team to meet that need.
4. Subdivide the allocation for each major category across the three levels of complexity until all boxes are filled (0% is an option). Vertical and horizontal percentages must sum appropriately. Example: If 30% of the group's needs fall into the category of health restoration, determine what portion of these needs are of high, medium, and/or low complexity, such as 20%, 5% and 5%, respectively.
5. (Optional; after Phase II) Estimate relative time requirements of activities per level of complexity. Do this by subdividing the percentage figure allocated to each category as follows: e.g., if 30% of patients' overall needs relate to health restoration, then decide how that figure of 30% should be subdivided across high-, medium-, and low-complexity activities to illustrate the proportionate workload related to each level.

a. Health care team—a multidisciplinary group of health care providers that intervene to meet the needs of a specific patient population.
b. See Table 12.3 for definitions of categories of patient needs.

redesign vision. The DSM finally provided a strategy to operationalize the expectation that new staff roles be based on patient needs rather than current task activity.

Second, it was initially believed that nursing could first identify the mix of nursing staff that would be required to meet a set of patient needs (MSEs, LPNs, and different levels of RNs) and then would be able to sit down with an interdisciplinary group to discuss overall staff activity for that population. That of course runs counter to a collaborative, futuristic paradigm. If nursing were to do the exercise independently, and in a manner that presupposed that they already knew what another profession could (or should) do, it would create unnecessary conflict.

Third, despite the above insight, it was at times necessary for nursing to use the differentiated staffing model for their own "unfreezing" purposes. In fact, one of the primary values of the tool has been to facilitate the ability of nurses to rethink nursing practice as it relates to the needs of patients; that is, how complex a particular need is and what a nurse, and a particular level of nurse, really should do to meet that need. The tool was particularly useful in helping staff to define for themselves which functions and components of care truly require a professional level of competency. Through this process, many nurses were for the first time explicitly identifying professional activities, such as critical thinking, assessment, collaboration, and coordination, in their daily practice. Some were beginning to see the difference in comparison to tasks such as medication administration and dressing changes. As one participant stated, "Once you use the model it is hard to get back to thinking about care in any other way." Another aspect of unfreezing was the need to let go of a valued task, such as teaching, that might well meet patient needs more effectively if provided at another point in the overall episode of care. In any case, while nurses were unfreezing paradigms about their own profession, it was still important not to allow them to make judgments for other disciplines.

Steps of the Model

The DSM presents a step-by-step format for critically reviewing (a) the comprehensive needs, per level of complexity, of a definable set of patients on a given unit; (b) the type of licensed and unlicensed personnel, across relevant disciplines, that could best meet those needs; and (c) the overall resultant staff mix that could deliver the needed care on that unit. More specifically:

- An interdisciplinary team identifies major homogeneous groupings of patients per a targeted unit or service (e.g., patients with leukemia). This team should include key professions that would traditionally be involved in such patients' care.

It also requires that the majority of group members have good clinical judgment and critical thinking skills, and be comfortable with conceptualization.

- This interdisciplinary team determines the nature of these patients' needs within the framework of health restoration, health maintenance, health promotion, environment, and coordination systems (see Table 12. 3). They judge the level of complexity and predictability of each of those categories of needs within the context of routine aspects of care (assessments, interventions, etc.).

- All needs are itemized so that the group is able to collectively "concretize" the concepts per category (see Table 12.4). As needs are thus identified and written for each category, they are evaluated as high (H), medium (M) or low (L) complexity. The discussion must include consideration of critical thinking and other complex aspects of practice, as with facets of assessment.

- The team now estimates the proportionate percentage of needs for each individual category, within relevant levels of complexity, for a grand total of 100%. It is important that the group thoroughly discuss and achieve consensus on their overall sense of the complexity of this set of needs. This is particularly true because there appears to be a tendency to overestimate complexity and to feel that each unit's group of patients is more complex than any other. This overestimation can lead to undervaluing important low- and medium-complexity components of care.

- The team next lists all of the roles/disciplines that could or should help to meet these diverse needs, per level of complexity (see Table 12.5). (In the actual DSM tool, separate pages are provided for high complexity, medium complexity, and low complexity. For Hartford, potential MSE roles were listed and, at this stage, only a generic RN role.) Each set of needs is then discussed, per level of need complexity, for the most appropriate role and level of expertise required. *Appropriate*, of course, relates to matching skill level of caregiver to the need of the patient; the lowest skill level is used within this criterion. An overall proportionate weight per role can finally be obtained from individual allocations.

- As part of the process, a running list of systems issues that can impede the delivery of care is kept for referral to management, but not discussed. Otherwise, these issues could invariably consume the majority of discussion time. Groups could also attempt to develop roles to meet system needs rather than patient needs.

- After the above activities, the Nursing group can now look at nursing positions and more definitively allocate activities within RN levels. They can also further define needed differentiation between RN versus LPN versus MSE.

- Following this initial allocation via complexity of needs, groups can go back and estimate the relative time requirements of the activities involved within each category. The unit of estimation is a percentage of the percentage figure allocated to that category: For example, if 30% of those patients' overall needs relate to health restoration, then how would that figure of 30% be subdivided across high-, medium-, and low-complexity activities to illustrate the proportionate workload related to each set of activities? Judgments are obviously only global but may eventually provide comparative time proportions among roles.

Table 12.6 provides a sample output from one differentiated staffing session that focused on a unit's respiratory population. In each box are two numbers separated by a diagonal line. The top number refers to the complexity and the bottom number to time as estimated in the last step. For example, it can be seen that for this population the needs cluster as either high or low complexity, with very few needs in between. The implications for role mix in such a case were primarily seen as a need for proficient/expert RNs, respiratory therapists, and multiskilled employees.

Reports on Use of the Model

As with many large-scale organizational projects similar to Patient-Centered Redesign, timelines established for various objectives have to be adjusted. One such objective was implementation of unit-based redesign to the extent that differentiation and other innovations would be fully implemented on targeted areas. Ultimate use of the model is now to be tested in the fall of 1993.

Despite this delay in its full use to date, the model has been tried with 14 different groups in one or another preliminary stage of change. Initial perceptions regarding the tool and related processes have been obtained through structured interviews with a representative sample of 10 small groups of head nurses, clinical nurse specialists, and/or nursing staff involved in the process. Several insights have thus been gained. Overall, although this information should be validated through a more rigorous evaluation process, the value of the DSM for Patient-Centered Redesign has been affirmed.

The types of units that used the model to at least some degree included hematology/oncology, obstetrics, cardiology (general and ICU), medicine, trauma, ortho, rehab, psychiatry, and surgery (general and ICU). The impetus for the DSM sessions varied. In a few cases, it was at the mandate of the nursing director ("initially [we did it] because we had to . . . then found out how useful the process is"). In most cases, however, nurse managers sought out the experience increasingly as they heard positive reports from peers. For example, one nurse manager was looking for a framework to facilitate a move to a new unit, which required a relook at staffing, and another wanted help "to change to meet changing patient care needs . . . to define new care needs" or to "help define the direction for patient care and assignments."

Approximately half of the sessions have used the model to rethink nursing. Sample participants in such cases included the nurse manager, assistant head nurse, selected staff nurses, and a clinical nurse specialist. The remainder of sessions to date have had multidisciplinary members—for example, nursing, pharmacy, social services, physical therapy, and/or respiratory. Some groups held multiple meetings. Each meeting is 1.5 hours in length, and at least three such meetings are needed to work through one group of patients. Some units, however, needed additional sessions because of the struggle to shed old paradigms: for example, through gradual realization of the need to view the population in the context of an entire episode of care rather than from one isolated unit's experience.

Overall, all those interviewed stated in one way or another that the process of working through the DSM served to change the way they looked at nursing and patient care. It helped them to identify what elements of care patients need and who should deliver those elements. It helped to operationalize the concept *patient-centered* and to break down "the basics of what patients need." As one interviewee stated, it "provided a means of looking at all the things that are done for patients and who really should be doing them." More specifically, some nurse managers and their staff learned to recognize elements of care that could be delegated. Some respondents were better able to differentiate professional from technical functions (and BSN from non-BSN) and to better understand the functions and role of other professions. The value of the tool is reflected in the following comments: "Refocused us; helped to redefine the work of nursing," and "There are many nonprofessional activities that could be performed by nonprofessional workers" (this was even true in an ICU group).

Specific goals that various groups had hoped to achieve through this process for the most part related to reviewing budgeted positions and related allocation of resources. Groups saw this tool as a way of identifying the type of workers they needed for a particular patient population in the context of cost containment and current health care issues. For example, one wanted "to deliver the same quality with fewer professionals . . . to help nurses do what they are prepared to do," and another "to come out with differentiated practice . . . to match patient needs with competency of staff and to look at the staffing mix." The extent to which these goals were met varied. Some did report making changes in budgeted positions, such as conversion of RN to patient care assistant (PCA) positions. The majority, however, indicated an increased delegation of tasks to existent PCAs and changes in how these assistants are assigned and used.

They also reported an increased emphasis on professional functions for the RN role:

- "Nurses are delegating more tasks now."
- "Those [staff] at the meetings learned that they can give some things away, that they don't have to do it all."

- "LPN assignments have changed. . . . RN now assigned as resource for LPN, with RN responsible for LPN functioning."
- "Have changed PCA assignment . . . working with the same nurses; staff involved now in hiring PCA and PCAs feel truly integrated in the team; staff developed PCA worksheet to enhance accountability."

The specific outcome that was least mentioned by these managers was differentiation within the RN role. This is a more difficult challenge, implicitly and inextricably connected with the always hot "BSN" and valuing issues. It also challenges old paradigms of how assignments are made and the belief of some that every RN should, a priori, be in the same role; for example, the expectations of some staff that every RN should be a "primary nurse" or case manager or PCC if he or she wants to, regardless of related competencies. Change and expectations such as true accountability and full implementation of unit-based redesign will obviously take more time. However, it should be noted that in leadership discussions, frequent comments regarding differentiation and use of "expert" nurses suggest a shift in paradigms. Gradual implementation of the role of the PCC (akin to a case manager's requiring higher level competencies) is also forcing the issue of differentiation within RNs.

Facilitating and Hindering Factors

As the process evolved, several potential facilitating and hindering factors were identified, in particular by the assistant project director responsible for conducting differentiated staffing sessions. Those that appeared to be facilitative included

1. *Involvement of the leader.* When the nurse manager supported the process, meetings were usually consistent and productive. The level of sophistication and ability of this individual to conceptualize the process, and herself unfreeze, were influential, and the value she placed on the process, not unexpectedly, was communicated to group members and in turn could affect their involvement.

2. *Selection of staff.* Meetings were more productive if staff were chosen for their clinical expertise, ability to think creatively and futuristically, and ability to negotiate ideas. To encourage selection of such a group, the facilitator would hold planning sessions with the nurse manager to carefully identify which staff optimally should be involved, rather than having automatic inclusion by "roles."

3. *Interdisciplinary focus.* Inclusion of other pertinent disciplines enhanced sharing of ideas and discussion. In such a group, participants were enabled to develop an awareness of each other's values and beliefs about professional patient care. One discipline could help another see components of care that could be delegated to multiskilled employees. Respiratory therapists, for example, identified that certain routine respiratory treatments could be delegated to an MSE, and social

workers identified elements of telephoning related to discharge planning that the unit secretary could assume.

4. *Use of an expert clinician.* An objective clinician, skilled in a specialty practice, enhanced the group's ability to look at a patient population creatively. Because of their clinical credibility, clinical nurse specialists were often able to reality-test old paradigms and encourage new thinking by staff—for example, regarding delegation of technical components of critical care.

5. *Use of a facilitator.* It is necessary that someone thoroughly understand the model before engaging staff or leadership. This individual needs process skills and must be comfortable allowing free flow in discussions and encouraging full participation.

Absence of the above factors—for example, selection of a negative, overbearing, or extremely resistant staff member—can of course be a hindrance. In addition, the following were also noted as adversely affecting differentiation sessions:

1. *Lack of follow-through.* If a nurse manager failed to follow through in terms of seeing that the same staff consistently got to meetings, there was a negative impact.

2. *Physicians.* Given their backgrounds, many physicians do not value process-related discussions, especially as detailed as these must be. Their input would most likely be more valuable in follow-up stages.

3. *Lack of clear goals and/or competing issues.* If a group has another agenda and/or is unclear as to the purpose of the session, difficulties will be encountered. Inability of the group to clearly identify their patient population can also interfere with the process. Microdefinition of patient groups was not found to be useful to the differentiation process.

4. *Individual versus group focus.* Early in the process, many groups became confused when considering patient needs because of frequently changing individual patient conditions. Discussion about laws of probability provided clarification. Groups were encouraged to consider the patient population "on average," knowing that all patients change over the course of an episode and that different patients in the same population will simultaneously be at different stages.

FINAL ISSUES AND SUMMARY

Large scale organizational change is often an incremental process. At a minimum, it can be said that at Hartford Hospital the differentiating staffing model has incrementally and successfully begun to affect old paradigms about nursing, staffing, and other disciplines. It has encouraged critical thinking about professional practice and facilitated dialogue between different disciplines not only about what a profession would like to contribute, but about what needs they are in a position to truly meet. It has provided a means to view the reallocation of activities among various roles, even to the point of suggesting that a specific role may no longer be cost-effective for a given population of patients.

The next challenge to the operationalization of differentiation will occur when a set of units implements unit-based redesign. To accomplish this, information gleaned from the DSM model (which includes the types and general proportions of a newly designed staff mix) must ultimately be converted into numbers. How many FTEs of each category will be needed to effectively and cost-efficiently meet the needs of a given population of patients must be projected. The previously described process of estimating time required for care-related needs has enabled some groups to see the balance among activity, complexity, and time required to perform components of care. This might be used to evolve future projections of types of staff and levels of workers; however, a great deal of work remains before a usable method is clarified. This task is a major challenge for several reasons:

- Hartford Hospital's acuity system is outdated and must be replaced; it cannot be "modified" to provided any meaningful data.
- Patient-Centered Redesign will continue to move forward with unit-based redesign prior to acquisition of a new system.
- Few, if any, current classification systems address a staffing mix from an interdisciplinary viewpoint.
- Many current systems focus too extensively on a laundry list of tasks and do not adequately address the workload nature of more complex professional behaviors such as collaborative care planning and outcomes assessment (see Prescott et al., 1991).

The future vision for Patient-Centered Redesign includes creation of an information system that can automatically track patient needs and their complexity and will enable the automatic identification of acuity based on those needs. In the meantime, decisions must be made about how many of the ideal staff mix should actually be put into a budget for redesigned units. Given time limitations, this process will in all likelihood utilize national HPPD standards for targeted populations, consideration of fiscal constraints, and the best judgment of leadership responsible for a given unit, within the context of the DSM. The hospital's management engineers, who are also now familiar with the principles and concepts of Patient-Centered Redesign and differentiation, can participate at this stage and, if possible, use computer simulation to map out potential staffing patterns. Such alternative methodologies must be considered because there is no ready formula to achieve the goal envisioned. In the end, the ideal mix must be converted into a 24-hour/7-day schedule. As such, it is expected that idealized redesign and several iterations may be needed until staff have learned how to more creatively and effectively meet the needs of patients through differentiation and interdisciplinary collaboration. As part of unit-based redesign, ongoing evaluation will enable revisions that are congruent with the principles of Patient-Centered Redesign and the framework of differentiation of nursing practice.

The National Strengthening Hospital Nursing Program frequently refers to the "spiraling journey" of organizational change. Implementation of differentiation at Hartford Hospital aptly fits that description as it has been incrementally advanced and continuously refined throughout the past 2 years. The differentiated staffing model has greatly facilitated that process by unfreezing old paradigms and introducing a new paradigm of patient-centered, cost-effective, interdisciplinary care. Progress in the next year may still not achieve the ultimate vision of differentiation, but because the profession of nursing has been struggling with this issue since at least 1965, miracles cannot be expected, and incrementalism can be considered a valid goal.

REFERENCES

Ackoff, R. L. (1981). *Creating the corporate future.* New York: John Wiley.

American Nurses Association. (Ed.). (1980). *Nursing: A social policy statement.* Kansas City, MO: Author.

Armstrong, D. M., & Stetler, C. B. (1991). Strategic considerations in developing a delivery model. *Nursing Economics, 9,* 112-115.

Benner, P. (1984). *From novice to expert: Excellence and power in clinical nursing practice.* New York: Addison-Wesley.

Goertzen, I. E. (1991). Preface. In I. E. Goertzen (Ed.), *Differentiating nursing practice into the twenty-first century* (pp. xi-xii). Kansas City, MO: American Academy of Nursing.

Hartford Hospital. (1990). *Strengthening Hospital Nursing Program.* In-house document.

Koerner, B., & Armstrong, D. (1983). Collaborative practice at Hartford Hospital. *Nursing Administration Quarterly, 7,* 72-81.

Kron, T., & Gray, A. (1987). *The management of patient care: Putting leadership skills to work* (6th ed.). Philadelphia: W. B. Saunders.

McClure, M. L. (1991). Introduction. In I. E. Goertzen (Ed.), *Differentiating nursing practice into the twenty-first century* (pp. 1-9). Kansas City, MO: American Academy of Nursing.

Milton, D., Verran, J., Murdaugh, C., & Gerber, R. (1991). Implementing differentiated practice as part of a professional practice model. In I. E. Goertzen (Ed.), *Differentiating nursing practice into the twenty-first century* (pp. 279-285). Kansas City, MO: American Academy of Nursing.

Murray, M. (1993). Where are the career ladders going in the 90's? *Nursing Management, 24*(6), 46-48.

National Program Office. (1992). *Strengthening hospital nursing: A program to improve patient care.* St. Petersburg, FL: Author.

Prescott, P., Ryan, J., Soeken, K., Castorr, A., Thompson, K., & Phillips, C. (1991). The patient intensity for nursing index: A validity assessment. *Research in Nursing and Health, 14*(3), 213-221.

Primm, P. L. (1987). Differentiated practice for ADN- and BSN-prepared nurses. *Journal of Professional Nursing, 3*(4), 218-224.

Wolahan, C. G. H. (1991). Differentiated practice: The competency model. In I. E. Goertzen (Ed.), *Differentiating nursing practice into the twenty-first century* (pp. 221-239). Kansas City, MO: American Academy of Nursing.

CHAPTER 13

The Colorado Differentiated Practice Model and Work Redesign

Marie E. Miller
Joyce L. Falco

The future holds many challenges for health care organiza-
tions. They will need to be innovative, diverse, and flexible in the delivery of
care in order to thrive in the marketplace. What an opportune time for nursing
to lead the way with the implementation of differentiated practice! The Colorado differentiated practice model for Nursing (CDPM) is being implemented
in six hospitals, four urban and two rural. These institutions are in the process
of redesigning the workplace to meet today's competitive challenges.

Similar to the U.S. Department of Health and Human Service
Secretary's Commission on Nursing in 1988, the Colorado Nursing Task Force
(1989) identified practice issues regarding patient care, work redesign, and
career advancement that affected nursing retention, recruitment and satisfaction. At the 22 public hearings held throughout Colorado, two issues pertaining
to the work environment were raised repeatedly by staff nurses. First, staff nurse
knowledge and expertise were not being sought, valued, and/or used to improve patient care due to lack of autonomy, participation, and input into the
system of care in institutions; and second, many staff nurses were not being
used to their full potential, in that their roles were identical regardless of
competency, education, and experience. The latter issue is linked to many

institutional factors such as staffing, job expectations, opportunity for variety and challenge within the work setting, and the need to develop and maximize one's abilities in the workplace. The development of the Colorado differentiated practice model (CDPM) addressed the concerns voiced by nurses through a reassessment of the roles and responsibilities of the different types of nurses and the work to be accomplished at the patient care level. Subsequent implementation of the CDPM redesigns the work of nurses in actual patient care systems such that the untapped potential of the nursing workforce is optimized through the use of committed, high-performing teams that transcend the collective potential of individual members. The evaluation component of the implementation project measures changes in patient and nurse variables before and after implementation to gauge the value of CDPM as a model to improve patient care and nurse satisfaction within the practice setting.

DIFFERENTIATED PRACTICE MODEL

The Colorado differentiated practice model for Nursing (1992) was developed by a task force of 200 staff nurses across the state. This unique model was developed to show how nursing education, competency, and experience interrelate in determining how a nurse may advance to a higher professional role while continuing to practice at the bedside. It is designed so that nurses with varying educational preparations and work experiences can most efficiently use their knowledge and skills while delegating non-nursing tasks to nurse extenders. Time spent by nurses on non-nursing tasks decreases the amount of time available for patient care activities and is not cost-effective. By varying the skill mix according to each unit's needs, a flexible, dynamic care delivery system that responds efficiently to the specific needs of each patient can be achieved. This model provides cost-effective nursing care that enables patients to have more input into their care and enhances nursing autonomy and accountability. Moreover, empowerment of nursing staff occurs as they take on new or expanded roles and are provided with ongoing education to continuously increase their expertise. Nurses are placed on separate clinical ladders based on their educational background: licensed practical nurse, associate degree/diploma RN, baccalaureate degree RN, nursing doctorate degree RN, and master's degree RN. The model incorporates competency statements and role descriptions, a clinical ladder, and pay-for-performance recommendations. It allows each nurse to advance and set his or her career goals on the basis of education, competency, and experience. As a long-term outcome, differentiated practice should promote unity in the profession in that it recognizes and rewards the unique contributions of all nurses, regardless of their educational

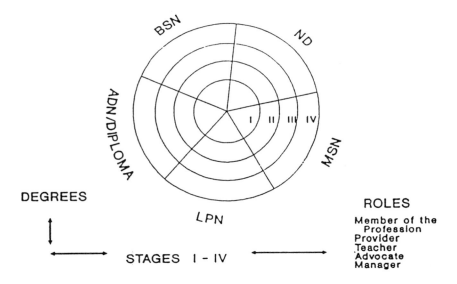

Figure 13.1. The Colorado Differentiated Practice Model for Nursing

background. This model also promotes respect and trust between all levels of nurses working together to achieve the common goal of delivering high-quality patient care. Figure 13.1 illustrates the multiple educational backgrounds, career stages, and nursing roles for staff nurses resulting in differentiated clinical practice. The model is circular to capture the wholeness of nursing practice and the varying contributions of all nurses at the bedside, based on education, competency, and experience. The model also incorporates the work of Benner (1984) and McBride (1985) in that it has four stages. Stage I depicts entry or beginning skill level, and the largest circle represents the expert or Stage IV nurse. Expert nurses at each educational level, depicted at the perimeter of the nursing system, influence all stages of nursing practice and are the primary interface with the broader health care system. The circles are intersected with five lines that meet in the center of the smallest to form five equal "slices." Each "slice" represents a level of nursing education and with its respective levels becomes the clinical ladder used for advancement that allows for pay-for-performance recommendations. The linear diagram at the bottom of the model depicts the five roles all nurses are expected to perform regardless of education and level of expertise. These roles become the foundation for leveling nursing skills and are Member of the Profession, Provider, Teacher, Advocate, and Manager. This model is driven by competency statements and role descriptions.

Implementation Process

Following development of the model, a call was issued to nursing practice sites in the state to determine interest in implementing the model. More than 60 institutions in the state requested consideration as an implementation site. Administrative support was solicited at each site before it was selected to be a pilot. Meetings with the chief executive officer and the director or vice president of Nursing were held to ensure their support of the project. Although the model was developed for use in a variety of practice settings, such as long-term care, hospitals, and home health care, the initial implementation is limited to hospitals and achieves a balance of urban and rural representation.

Institutional Structures. Each of the six pilot sites is choosing to implement the model using different strategies. The two rural sites are implementing the model hospital-wide. Two urban hospitals, under the same corporate umbrella, are implementing it on two units at each site that have recently implemented work redesign, a third urban site is piloting it on one unit, and the last site has chosen to implement it at the time of starting up a new six-bed neurotrauma unit. The sites that recently implemented work redesign are attempting to fully utilize human resources, as again use of this model facilitates by recommending that the "right nurse do the right job." In implementation of differentiated practice, just as with work redesign, both the technical and social aspects of the system are optimized. At each of the six pilot sites, a coordinator was selected who would work on the project approximately one-quarter time, with the project coordinator, who was assigned full time to rotate among the sites. Two of the site coordinators are the nurse managers on units doing the implementation, one is a house supervisor, one is a staff nurse, one is the education director, and one is a special projects coordinator.

A Clinical Ladder Committee and an Education Committee have been set up in each site to assist with implementation. Both committees have been empowered to incorporate the unique values and culture critical to accomplishing the goals of the model in their particular institution. The size of the committees varies from site to site, with as few as 2 to as many as 18 members. Both groups met twice per month during the first year with the project and site coordinators. On the basis of the experience of Sioux Falls Hospital in implementing the CDPM (Koerner, Bunkers, Nelson, & Santema, 1989), participating staff nurses were provided with information and education to facilitate the process. Conferences at the sites documented that staff need education to implement this change successfully and to become empowered to take on new roles. Therefore, the goals of the Education Committee were to plan, organize, and coordinate the development and delivery of the educational modules to facilitate the process in each site. This was accomplished by meeting the following objectives: (a) develop a format for the educational modules, with emphasis on the content, teaching and learning strategies, and delivery methods; (b) develop procedures for evaluating the effectiveness of the educational modules; (c) develop a schedule for delivery of the educational modules and a process for monitoring completion of the educational modules for all participating nurses; (d) develop educational materials to be included in educational workbooks on each module; (e) conduct ongoing evaluation process; and (f) deliver educational modules to other hospital personnel and administrators.

The meeting schedule of the Clinical Ladder Committees was the same; however, they met more hours per month to achieve their goals. The objectives for the Clinical Ladder Committee were to (a) develop skills checklists for each participating unit; (b) incorporate the institutional goals into the performance evaluation; (c) develop the professional activities list as a component of the clinical ladder; (d) develop position descriptions and performance evaluations based on the competency statements in the model for each of the educational levels of nurses participating at their site; and (e) develop policies and procedures for administering and managing the clinical ladder in each site—placement of nurses, peer review, and advancement policies. In addition to the individual site meetings, representatives from each committee have come together to meet once per quarter to discuss issues and to learn from each other how the process is working in each site. Site coordinators have met together with the project director, coordinator, and manager on a quarterly basis for problem solving and to provide direction and timelines. During the second year of implementation, the committees will combine and meet formally once per month with the project and site coordinators to ensure the smooth implementation of the model in the workplace.

Education Program. The Education Committees defined the educational needs of the staff nurses and recommended that 12 modules be developed. These modules will enable staff to develop new skills or to build upon existing skills to enhance team cohesiveness. On the work redesign units, self-directed teams are being formed, and the team members are being educated about both work redesign and differentiated practice and the interrelationship of these concepts. The modules are (a) Overview of the Colorado Differentiated Practice Model for Nursing; (b) Most Frequently Asked Questions About the Colorado Differentiated Practice Model; (c) Focus on the Competency Statements and the Colorado Differentiated Practice Model; (d) Change Process; (e) Myer-Briggs Type Indicator®; (f) Organizational Culture; (g) Group Process; (h) Team Building; (i) Conflict Resolution; (j) Communication Techniques; (k) The

Colorado Differentiated Practice Model for Each Institution; and (1) Marketing Yourself. The committees contributed to the development of the modules along with consultants and project staff. The modules consist of a videotape (filmed at the Media Resource Center at the University of Colorado Health Sciences Center) using project staff and consultants, and a workbook containing 12 chapters, to correlate with each video; each chapter contains learner objectives and activities, a content outline of the video, and a bibliography. Each participating nurse has received a workbook that can be referred to whenever necessary. The nurses earn continuing education credit for each module completed, and they are expected to complete all of them, either in the group sessions held at each site or on an individual basis. The committee planned specific learning activities for the nurses to complete following each video presentation. The videos range from 35 to 60 minutes in length and the activities another 30 to 45 minutes. At each site, the Education Committee members developed their teaching, facilitation, and leadership skills. Through this strategy, the project builds self-sustaining capacity within the institution for the future. Each facility has its own copies of all 12 videos so that as new staff are hired, they can be introduced to differentiated practice.

Clinical Ladder. The Clinical Ladder Committee at each site developed position descriptions and performance evaluations based on components of the clinical ladder: competency statements for each educational level across each of the four stages, a professional activities lists, skill checklists, and institutional goals. Although the model dictates the competency statements, institutions develop their own skill checklists, professional activities list, and institutional goals. Currently, each Clinical Ladder Committee is developing policies and procedures for administering and managing the clinical ladder in each site—that is, peer review and advancement procedures for both stages and levels. At the end of 1 year, nurses will have an opportunity for movement on the clinical ladder based on their performance as well as their desire to do so. Now that each site is working with various components of the clinical ladder—competency statements, professional activities list, skills checklists, and institutional goals—we expect that revisions will be needed. The competency statements by educational category and stage are being evaluated by all participating staff nurses in the pilot project. As we find through work redesign what works and what does not, the CDPM will be refined and rewritten to incorporate the necessary changes for implementation on a broader scale.

Placement on the Model. At each site, initial placement and validation of the placement of participating nurses took place. The placement procedure varied

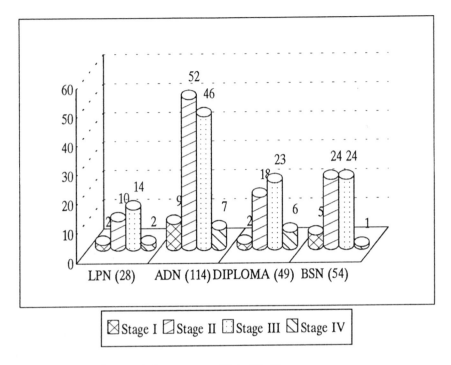

Figure 13.2. Staff Nurses' Placement on Clinical Ladders

at the sites, with some choosing self-placement only and others choosing a combination of self-placement and nurse manager placement. Nurses initially placed themselves on the ladder according to how they evaluated themselves with regard to the competency statements. There are four stages: Stage I, entry level nurse; Stage II, competent nurse; Stage III, highly proficient nurse; and Stage IV, expert nurse. Nurses choose which stage they practice in, because this is a model based on self-pacing and career choice.

At meetings during the model's development, the group predicted that the distribution of nurses across the stages of each educational level would be likely to approximate a normal distribution, with the majority of nurses falling in Stages II and III of the model. This hypothesis led to the development of four levels in Stages II and III and two levels in Stages I and IV, for a total of 12 levels on the clinical ladder for each educational category. Figure 13.2 shows the initial placement of a sample of 266 nurses from all six sites on their respective clinical ladders by stage with the majority falling in Stages II and III. Thus the preliminary data support the predicted distribution pattern. Note that there are no nursing doctorate (ND) or master's degree RN placements, because currently no nurses are practicing at the bedside in any of the pilot sites.

Accreditation. The Joint Commission on Accreditation of Healthcare Organizations (JCAHO, 1991) recommended the use of differentiated practice models for nursing in its guidelines for nursing care standards:

> Health care delivery organizations should adopt innovative nurse staffing patterns that recognize and appropriately utilize the different levels of education, competence, and experience among registered nurses, as well as between registered nurses and other nursing personnel responsible to registered nurses, such as licensed practical nurses and ancillary personnel (Relevant Required Characteristics: NC.3.4.2, NC.3.4.2.1). (p. 17)

The CDPM embodies the same principles of differentiation among and between registered nurses and practical nurses using education, experience, and competence as in the JCAHO recommendation. The JCAHO guidelines further recommended assessing competencies consistently with the process contained in the CDPM clinical ladder concept:

> *Assessment of competence.* The knowledge and skills required to competently provide hospital-based nursing care are constantly changing based on advances in patient care techniques and technology and increases in patients' severity of illness. The Task Force therefore believed that the need to accurately assess the competence of individual nursing staff members (and to assign them patient care responsibilities accordingly) is increasingly important. (New Required Characteristics NC.2.1 through NC.2.1.2.2.2 pertain to evaluation of competence using information from a variety of sources.) (p. 19)

The new nursing care standards support continuous improvement in quality. Monitoring and evaluation of the nursing staff are key components of the process. This requires rethinking the work of nursing in light of new technologic advances in patient care and the relationship of nursing to other aspects of the health care delivery system. It will require nursing to periodically examine and redesign the sociotechnical aspects of the nursing care delivery system.

WORK REDESIGN

General definitions of work redesign describe a process of employee participation in rethinking the way work gets done. Additional expected outcomes associated with work redesign are responsibility, accountability, job enrichment, empowerment, heightened commitment to the work unit, and increased identification with the organization. Early work redesign efforts drew from Japanese-style management practices; however, more recent advances tend toward quality-of-work-life approaches. Relevant elements in the latter approach include the technical and social environment within the organization as well as the administrative system and the relationship between life at work and other aspects of one's life (Cunningham & Eberle, 1990). Quality-of-work-life designs develop from understanding the needs of the technology as well as the social needs of the individuals in the system. This approach requires a commitment from administration to understand the problems and adopt appropriate techniques to support the redesign effort, including the involvement of staff in the redesign process and reasonable attempts to facilitate staff implementation of the final model.

In differentiated practice, work redesign begins with initial rethinking of the nursing organization at the patient care level. At some sites this initial step has served as the catalyst for more comprehensive rethinking of patient care delivery by other departments in collaboration with nursing or as a springboard for implementing more comprehensive work redesign efforts involving many departments within the institution. At other sites it is limited to the nursing units. Staff participate in a comprehensive analysis, examining the technical, social, and managerial aspects of nursing care delivery. Unit teams envision the work of nursing in light of the CDPM, the patient caseload, the mix of nursing staff, and the desired outcomes in order to redesign nursing roles and responsibilities that optimize the full potential of team members. The nature of tasks, skill levels, knowledge bases, norms, clinical outcomes, supervision, and patient care management are considered in structuring role responsibilities and configurations. As implementation progresses, nursing staff redesign their traditional ways of working together to optimize the utilization of each educational category of worker on the basis of patient needs and the technical aspects of the care. Work redesign must meet both the technical requirements of the tasks and the social/psychological requirements of the workers to be successful in improving the effectiveness and efficiency of the unit.

Donovan (1989) stated that the goal of redesign "is to develop an organization that optimizes both the technical and social aspects of the system," and he further identified the self-directing team as the building block of a redesigned work system. A self-directing team is one that takes responsibility and accountability for planning, controlling, and doing all of the work needed for its portion of the business, including managing performance, safety, quality, and efficiency. Differentiated nursing practice enables the formation of self-directed work teams on the units by affirming the different but complementary knowledge and skills that each educational type brings to the work environment. The model assumes that the most appropriate person will be called upon to bring his or her expertise to bear on the patient's problems. At some sites bacca-laureate-prepared nurses serve as case managers on nursing teams so that their expertise brings a broader perspective to patient care. Others have imple-mented multiskilled assistants to decrease the non-nursing tasks of the nursing staff. And some have requested new hires with specific knowledge and skills to complement the existing staff, using the CDPM to recommend a particular category of nurse.

The competencies in the model help the team to reconceptualize nursing roles and relationships. Rigorous debate emerges from the nursing staff as they reexamine assumptions, attitudes, and current nursing practice. Sometimes during the process, teams will suspend assumptions and enter a genuine dis-cussion period of "thinking together" as Senge (1990) described. Delegation practices, for example, generate complex discussion and engage some teams in exceptionally productive analysis of specific tasks, including training, policies, supervision, and performance aspects, resulting in renegotiated role responsi-bilities. These discussions are essential to the redesign process for the work to become the responsibility of the group and for the planning and assignment aspects to be incorporated within the team's control. They also foster en-trepreneurship within the team. If the team know what they need to be more successful, if they have (or can obtain) the resources to do it, and if they are able to act, they will take control to get the job done right. Self-directed teams are indispensable components of the continuous quality improvement desired by all institutions.

On a practical level, a self-directed team increases the number of problems that can be handled simultaneously by the team and increases its ownership of problems and outcomes. Structural barriers are reduced, and group learning can occur at an exponential rate facilitated by the communication and relation-ship aspects of team behavior. In addition, the model increases the alignment of goals between the staff and management and decreases the need for man-agement oversight. The staff share the same vision, values, and goals as manage-ment as they incorporate the institution's goals into their performance plans for the clinical ladder. Improvement and excellence are bred as the staff direct themselves to pursue through individual and team efforts goal areas to work on that are priorities for their practice area and unit. The institutional goals and professional activities areas of the career ladder component of the model provide a menu for focusing professional growth and development consistent with individual, team, and institutional priorities. Team members elevate and expand their thinking to the system level as they are challenged to rethink their work in relation to the whole.

HUMAN RESOURCES

Dialogue with Human Resource representatives from each site began early on. Because this model recommends pay for performance, it is essential that the Human Resource Department from each site be included in the implementation process. Some issues of concern are that the model is complex, does not fit traditional current compensation models, may not fit the hospital compensation package, and may further compress salaries. During the first year of implementation, nurses will receive salary adjustments based on the current system in their institution. If we can show during the second year that nurses do indeed practice differently—for example, BSNs performing the case manager role—then "a nurse is a nurse is a nurse" is not true, and there will be a stronger case for pursuing the pay-for-performance recommendations outlined for the second year. An organization's ability to change job descriptions, pay and reward systems, training and recruitment mechanisms, and group management practices enters into the debate on these issues.

Differentiated practice and work redesign presuppose a change in philosophy of organization and corresponding job involvement, including changes in classification and a changing management approach. Also, differentiated practice provides objective measures for advancement in an evolving professional model with recognition and reward. However, compatibility with the organization is essential, and the nursing clinical ladder will have to be integrated within the larger system. Salary considerations encompass the following:

- Establishing the salary range from entry to expert for each educational category
- Establishing a different job description for each educational category with different expectations and titles
- Comparing current salaries with projected salaries if CDPM recommendations are implemented
- Evaluating the compression effect of stages and levels
- Projecting the short-term and long-term cost impact on the pilot units, and extrapolating those figures to the Nursing Department

The hospitals in the pilot project were already engaged in the change process before CDPM. This facilitated integration of differentiated practice and work redesign within the institution because an openness to innovation was present. Dialogue between nursing administration and Human Resources in terms of restructuring the work force was ongoing. Salary costs are an issue of great concern to all health care institutions; the collaborative efforts of Human Resources and nursing administration are essential to establishing the pay and reward structure for the CDPM.

TABLE 13.1   Framework for Evaluation of the Colorado Differentiated Practice
              Model for Nursing

Pilot Program	Impact 1	Impact 2	Outcome
Components	Predisposing Factors	Nurse Teams	Decreased
Program	Institutional	Education sessions	Turnover
Structure	philosophy	Work redesign	Costs per patient day
Administration	Administrative	Enact model	
	support	Evaluate model	
		Refine model	
	Enabling Factors		Increased
	Resources		Work satisfaction
	Site Coordinator		Patient satisfaction
	Placement on ladder		Group cohesion
			Productivity
	Reinforcing Factors		
	Education Committee		
	Clinical Ladder Com-		
	Committee		
Input variables	Intervening variables	Process variables	Outcome variables

EVALUATION

The primary question of importance for the pilot sites (or for any institution that chooses to implement the CDPM) is whether there is a return on investment: Will the investment of resources result in benefits for the organization? The evaluation framework for the CDPM (Table 13.1) outlines the broad categories of variables and specifies the presumed causal relationships between categories of variables. The pilot program imposes the model, a structure for implementation, and external administration. Predisposing factors of philosophy and administrative support are essential for implementation. Other enabling and reinforcing factors intervene in the process of implementing the model with the nurse teams. The framework is designed to evaluate the impact on specific outcomes believed to be indicators of improved patient care, work conditions, and nurse retention.

A framework for evaluation expedites the selection of measures and instrument construction (Green & Lewis, 1986). It can help determine whether relevant instruments exist with tested reliability and validity to meet the requirements of the study or whether some need to be constructed. It provides a structure to guide the staging and level of analysis along with the specificity and scope of the evaluation.

Analysis is at the individual and aggregate level, with data collection points before and after implementation. The set of measures collected for the institution includes unit staffing mix, patient readmissions, operating expenses per patient day, turnover rate, supplemental staffing costs, overtime costs, and staff salary data. Nurses complete a demographic profile, Index of Work Satisfaction (Stamps & Piedmonte, 1986), Professional Identify Index (Brenner, 1986), Group Cohesion Scale (Good & Nelson, 1973), and assessment of the education program. Patients complete a newly constructed satisfaction questionnaire. Along with the quantitative analysis, extensive field notes are compiled for all of the meetings. We anticipate that this documentation will be a rich resource for future site implementation.

CONCLUSIONS

This model was developed by Colorado nurses with four basic goals. First, its ultimate focus is to improve patient care by promoting the use of the right nurse for the right job. Second, it redesigns the work of nursing to optimize the utilization of nursing education, competency, and experience in a way that values and respects the contribution of all types of nursing personnel. Third, it promotes a professional model of nursing practice that will retain nurses and nursing expertise at the bedside where they are desperately needed. Finally, it compensates nurses on the basis of their contribution to patient care. Thus far, pilot implementation of the model has empowered nursing staff by involving them in process improvement, problem solving, and decision making to improve patient care and nursing practice. As a result, they are better able to articulate nursing roles through examination and reflection on role components. This is a path of innovation and change that health care institutions need to consider seriously to compete in the declining market share and shrinking reimbursement dollars of the managed care marketplace.

REFERENCES

Benner, P. (1984). *From novice to expert.* Reading, MA: Addison-Wesley.
Brenner, P. S. (1986). Temporal perspective, professional identity, and perceived well being (Doctoral dissertation, Wayne State University). *Dissertation Abstracts International, 47,* 4821B.
Colorado Differentiated Practice Model for Nursing. (1992). Denver: Colorado Nursing Task Force.
Colorado Nursing Task Force. (1989). *Task force on nursing recommendations.* Denver, CO: Author.
Cunningham, J. B., & Eberle, T. (1990, February). A guide to job enrichment and redesign. *Personnel,* 56-61.
Donovan, M. (1989, December). Redesigning the workplace. *Journal for Quality and Participation,* (Suppl.), 6-8.
Good, L. R., & Nelson, D. A. (1973). Effects of person-group and intragroup attitude similarity on perceived group attractiveness and cohesiveness. *Psychological Reports, 33,* 551-560.

Green, L. W., & Lewis, F. M. (1986). *Measurement and evaluation in health education and health promotion.* Palo Alto, CA: Mayfield.

Joint Commission on Accreditation of Healthcare Organizations. (1991). *An introduction to Joint Commission Nursing Care standards.* Chicago: Author.

Koerner, J. E., Bunkers, L. B., Nelson, B., & Santema, K. (1989, February). Implementing differentiated practice: The Sioux Valley Hospital experience. *Journal of Nursing Administration, 19*(2), 13-20.

McBride, A. (1985, September/October). Orchestrating a career. *Nursing Outlook, 33*(5), 244-247.

Senge, P. (1990). *The fifth discipline.* New York: Doubleday.

Stamps, P. L., & Piedmonte, E. (1986). *Nurses and work satisfaction. An index for measurement.* Ann Arbor: Health Administration Press Perspectives.

CHAPTER 14

Reorganizing Hospital Nursing Resources: A Self-Managed Unit Model

Dorothy L. Gordon
Carol S. Weisman
Sandra D. Cassard
Rebecca Wong

New models of nursing practice are being developed in response to major forces of change in the health care environment. A self-managed unit model of professional nursing practice has been in operation at the Johns Hopkins Hospital for over 10 years. Based on concepts found in organization, human relations, and nursing literature, the model was designed to improve nursing satisfaction and retention as well as quality of care. This chapter presents the conceptual basis of the model and results of an evaluation of its effectiveness in relation to nurses' work satisfaction and retention, patient outcomes, and costs. Implications for nursing and hospital administrators are discussed.

Hospital environments changed dramatically in the 1980s, and continued change is inevitable in the future as health care is redirected to prevention, primary care, and outpatient and home health services. Hospital

AUTHORS' NOTE: Research reported in this chapter was funded by the National Institute for Nursing Research, National Institutes of Health, NR02091, 1989-1993. We gratefully acknowledge the collaboration in this project of our late colleague, Marilyn Bergner, PhD, of the Johns Hopkins School of Hygiene and Public Health.

and nursing administrators, however, will continue to be challenged to deliver quality patient care in a cost-effective environment while retaining competent professional nurses who have numerous employment options.

To meet this challenge, a wide variety of approaches to reorganizing nursing practice have been initiated (Rose & DiPasquale, 1990). Some are innovative attempts to bring modern management concepts and psychosocial principles of job design to patient care units. In an overview of selected nursing practice models, Weisman (1991) described them as differing from traditional models in the following characteristics:

1. The degree to which the practice of the individual nurses is differentiated according to education level or performance competencies.
2. The degree to which nursing practice at the unit level is self-managed, rather than managed by traditional supervisors.
3. The degree to which case management is employed.
4. The degree to which teams, either nursing or multidisciplinary, are employed.

Many practice models contain more than one of these elements and also include elements of primary nursing. One such innovative model has been in place at the Johns Hopkins Hospital (JHH) for 13 years and involves self-managing nursing units.

At JHH as well as other institutions, the impetus for creating new approaches to organizing nursing practice was rooted in the cyclical shortages of professional nurses and the failure of traditional administrative remedies, which view shortages as supply-side contractions. In that situation, hospital strategy concentrates on raising salaries to attract more of the available nurses. The nature of the hospital nursing shortage in the late 1970s and 1980s, however, was concluded to be the result of a demand for more nurses due to increased patient acuity, shorter hospital lengths of stay, increased technology, and an aging population. It was compounded by decreased enrollment in schools of nursing (U.S. Department of Health and Human Services, 1988). Accordingly, attention began to shift to strategies for increasing retention and utilizing nursing resources more effectively, in addition to recruitment.

With administrative and consultative support in 1980, one head nurse and a team of nurses at JHH designed a new professional practice model (PPM) that was implemented on one neurosurgical unit and had diffused to 16 units by 1990. (No unit that has adopted the PPM has discontinued it.) Its objectives were to increase work satisfaction and reduce job turnover among professional nurses. Operationally, the model is implemented via an informal contract between nurses and administration wherein the nurses agree to provide 24-hour nursing care for a year to the patients on their unit in exchange for unit self-management, salaries (as opposed to hourly wages), and gain sharing.

THE SETTING

Johns Hopkins Hospital is a private not-for-profit hospital affiliated with a major academic medical center in Baltimore, Maryland. There were 1,522 registered nurse (RN) FTEs at the 979-bed hospital in fiscal year 1991, with an RN-to-bed ratio of 1.6 to 1. The institution's management system is decentralized, with 10 operating clinical departments reporting to the hospital president. Each is headed by a physician chief to whom a nursing director and administrator report. Within the departments, each nursing unit has a nurse manager (head nurse) who holds authority and responsibility for its operations. Primary nursing is in place throughout the institution. A vice president for Nursing holds overall accountability for standards and quality of nursing practice and care, compensation, and professional development. The nursing directors have operational responsibility for their departments. Nurse managers are responsible for their unit's personnel budget planning and management and for monitoring supply budgets.

Monthly meetings are held between the nursing vice president and directors of Nursing for communication, coordinating, planning, and evaluation, and the vice president also meets regularly with the nurse managers.

CONCEPTUAL AND OPERATIONAL DIMENSIONS

Human resources and organizational nursing literature related to job design and self-managing work groups provide the conceptual basis of the PPM. Job design restructures the work environment and job characteristics to enhance employees' work experience and/or improve productivity. It is a method of improving organizational effectiveness. Because jobs do not occur in isolation within complex organizations, it is important that the setting and assumptions of the administration and workers be considered. Decentralization is a hallmark of JHH's organizational culture, and authority for decision making has been delegated to the organizational level where needed. Any model considered, therefore, would have to be compatible with such an environment. Similarly, professional nursing practice is highly valued, so that two assumptions were considered in planning the PPM: (a) registered nurses perceive themselves as professionals and, accordingly, strive to control their practice and expect to satisfy higher needs in the workplace (Weisman, 1982), and (b) registered nurses are career oriented, and a predominant orientation among

TABLE 14.1   Conceptual and Operational Aspects of the Johns Hopkins Hospital
Nursing Professional Practice Model (PPM)

Identified Source of Job Dissatisfaction[a]	Corresponding Job/ Organizational Context Characteristic[b]	Corresponding Change Strategy of PPM[c]	Operational Aspects of PPM[d]
Degree of control over work content and process; decision latitude	Autonomy	Participative decision making	Typically enacted by committees on the unit and include, at a minimum, staffing/scheduling, quality assurance, and peer review
Task routinization; inability to use skills	Skill variety; task identity	Primary nursing	Primary nursing
Opportunities for professional development, career advancement, and earning potential	Feedback; rewards and incentives	Unit peer review; upgraded pay level; salaried registered nurse staff	Typically includes peer feedback on performance and adherence to group defined rules; annual salaries; gain sharing

a. As identified by Dear, Weisman, and O'Keefe (1985).
b. As described in the job design and human resource management literature.
c. Incorporated into the PPM.
d. Each PPM unit develops a unit self-management agreement that is negotiated with the director of Nursing on an annual basis.

hospital staff nurses is toward a "linear" career involving advancement within the field (Friss, 1982). Change strategies at JHH therefore included redesigning nurses' jobs for greater unit-level control and structuring career pathways for nurses in the hospital within a decentralized organization.

Table 14.1 displays the conceptual and structural basis for the JHH PPM. Numerous research reports revealed dissatisfaction among nurses at JHH and other organizations related to dimensions of their jobs and organizational matters (Kramer, 1974; Price & Mueller, 1981; Weisman, Alexander, & Chase, 1981). These major sources of nurses' job dissatisfaction and turnover fell into three groupings: degree of control over work content and process and nurses' decision latitude at work; degree of task routinization and nurses' inability to use their skills in practice; and degree of responsibility for professional development and career advancements (Dear, Weisman, & O'Keefe, 1985).

The sources of job dissatisfaction relate to key job or organizational dimensions described by Hackman and Oldham (1976). These salient features of work include: autonomy (or the degree to which workers control their scheduling and work procedures); skill variety (or the degree to which the job requires workers to perform a variety of tasks or operations in performing their work); task identity (or the degree to which workers complete a "whole" piece of work and can identify outcomes of their work); and feedback (or the degree to which the job provides information to the worker about his or her performance). Jobs perceived as scoring higher on these dimensions are expected to produce critical "psychological states" (experienced responsibility for outcomes of work, knowledge of the actual results of work activities, and experienced meaningfulness of the work) (Hackman & Lawler, 1971; Hackman & Oldham, 1976). Higher levels of these states are expected, in turn, to positively influence the employee's internal work motivation, quality of work performance, satisfaction with work, and attendance behavior (Sethi, Berkwood, & Schuler, 1989).

Therefore, specific change strategies or interventions to redesign each problem area were the basis of the PPM. For example, participative decision making (autonomy) is implemented through self-management and operationalized through committees on the unit. Although any number of committees exist within any individual nursing unit, and are reflective of each unit's unique nature, all must include staffing/scheduling, quality assurance, and peer review. Unit scheduling committees, for example, can design their own shift system, assign people to shifts, develop an on-call system, or oversee a self-scheduling approach. The nurses, however, are themselves totally responsible for providing 24-hour coverage every day of the year. PPM nurses have input into setting and managing staffing levels.

Primary nursing (skill variety and task identity) is a key strategy in the PPM and already was in place when redesign was initiated. A primary nurse holds 24-hour responsibility and accountability for a patient's nursing care plan throughout his or her length of stay and has increased decision-making authority. A variety of professional nursing skills are required in comparison to traditional nursing care management, and the nurse has the opportunity to evaluate the patient's outcome in relation to the professional process of care. As compared to other modes of care (e.g., team or functional), primary nursing is generally thought to contribute to the enrichment of nursing jobs (Alexander, Weisman, & Chase, 1981). Within the PPM, features of primary nursing such as continuity and coordination were structurally reinforced. The change strategy related to "feedback" was the institution of unit-level peer review, which is thought to modify work-related behavior. Nurses utilize peer review in relation to performance standards and adherence to their operating guidelines.

Salaries as opposed to hourly wages were implemented to enhance professionalism and to provide rewards to foster long-term career orientation. Pay levels were upgraded by 10% over the base for each position level to compensate nurses for foregone overtime and shift differentials, as well as additional management tasks. Gain sharing was instituted in which nurses on model units share any year-end savings in unit labor costs with the hospital and as a group determine their distribution and/or use. This important component theoretically acts as an incentive to provide care with a leaner RN staff and fewer temporary personnel.

The operational aspects of a unit's PPM are delineated in an annual written agreement with the director of Nursing. When a group of registered nurses wish to implement the PPM on their unit, they develop the philosophy and objectives of the model on their unit, develop nursing care and practice standards, define roles and relationships of group members within the group, and define the structure and procedures for implementation.

The development of the model on a unit by a group of nurses, the annual commitment by members of the group to provide and manage nursing care according to the agreement, and the monitoring of its overall performance by the group itself reflect the idea of the JHH PPM as a self-managed work group. As defined in the literature (Goodman, Davadas, & Hughson, 1988), such a group is composed of individuals "who can self regulate work on their interdependent tasks" (p. 296). They differ from co-acting groups, in which people work close to one another on individually defined tasks, in that the work belongs to the group as a whole and the work group is the basic performing unit of the organization (Hackman & Oldham, 1980; Sethi et al., 1989). Self-managing work groups are expected to be more effective in part because group synergy creates efficiencies in the work process (Hackman & Oldham, 1980).

The opportunity for employees to participate fully in the management of work is expected to increase worker satisfaction as well as improve the group's productivity and effectiveness. Three dimensions of group effectiveness described by Hackman (1990) are the degree to which the group's service is acceptable to those who receive it; the degree to which the process of working together on a task improves the capability of future interdependent work among group members; and the degree to which the teamwork fosters individual group members growth and well-being. These dimensions relate to objectives of the PPM. Patients receive and evaluate nursing care, retention must be present for future group performance, and work satisfaction is one aspect of personal well-being.

EVALUATION OF THE PPM

A comprehensive evaluation of the effects of the PPM on nurses' work satisfaction and retention, on patients' satisfaction and outcomes, and on unit costs was conducted in 1990-1992 with funding from the National Institute for Nursing Research. The evaluation research took explicit recognition of the fact that although the PPM had been designed primarily to improve nurses' work satisfaction and retention, its possible effects on patient care and on unit costs were of considerable interest to both nursing and hospital management. On the basis of the theory cited earlier and an earlier evaluation (Dear et al., 1985), the PPM was hypothesized to increase nurses' work satisfaction and retention, to improve patient satisfaction and patient outcomes, and to reduce unit costs.

This evaluation occurred at a time when 16 nursing units at JHH had been using the PPM for at least 2 years. Because nursing units were self-selected to the PPM, a matched-unit design was used to assess PPM effects. However, only 8 of the 16 PPM units could be matched with traditionally managed (TM) units in the same general clinical area and with approximately the same RN staff size. Nevertheless, the evaluation contains a larger number of self-managed units in more clinical areas than have previously been studied. The clinical areas included are general medical, surgical, and pediatrics units; general operating rooms; and critical care units.

The evaluation used multiple methods of data collection. Table 14.2 summarizes the study variables, measures, and findings. To assess effects of the PPM on nurses' work satisfaction and retention, a survey of staff RNs on the eight PPM units and eight matched TM units was conducted using self-administered questionnaires, and retention was monitored for 12 months following the survey. Interviews were conducted with the nurse manager of each study unit. To assess the effects of the PPM on patients, a patient satisfaction survey was administered to a case series of eligible patients on the day of discharge from the study units. To assess the effects of the PPM on patient outcomes, a telephone interview was conducted with the same patients 2 weeks post discharge to measure perceived health status, perceived functional status, unmet needs for care, and unplanned health care utilization. In addition, hospital records were used to measure readmissions within 31 days of discharge, unit length of stay, diagnoses, patient severity of illness at admission to the unit, and unit costs.

With regard to PPM effects on nurses' work satisfaction and retention, results of the evaluation were positive (Weisman, Gordon, Cassard, Bergner, & Wong, 1993). Nurses on PPM units were found to have both higher work satisfaction levels and higher retention levels than nurses on TM units. In multivariate analyses, the positive impact of the PPM on work satisfaction was found to operate through two work process variables: improvements in co-ordination of patient care and more effective team performance, as perceived

TABLE 14.2 Major Outcome Variables Studied and Summary of Results

Type of Outcome	Key Measures	Significant Effects of PPM
Nursing outcomes	Work satisfaction	$+$[a]
	Retention (over 1 year)	$+$[b]
Patient outcomes	Satisfaction on day of discharge	0
	Perceived health and functional status on day of discharge	0
	Unplanned health care utilization during 2 weeks post discharge	0
	Hospital readmission within 31 days of discharge	0
	Unmet ADL and IADL needs during 2 weeks post discharge	0
Unit costs	Nursing personnel expenditures (employees and purchased nursing services)	Mixed[c]
	Recruitment and orientation costs	Inadequate data

a. PPM is associated with higher nurses' work satisfaction.
b. PPM is associated with higher nurse retention.
c. PPM is associated with lower expenditures for nursing in inpatient units and with higher expenditures in ORs.

by the nurses. The impact of the PPM on retention appears to be indirect, through its positive effect on work satisfaction.

Furthermore, PPM nurses were found to work longer hours than comparison nurses (in part due to the requirement of on-call time) and to earn higher pay; longer hours reduced work satisfaction in multivariate analyses, but higher pay increased retention. These contradictory effects of the PPM need to be taken into account when implementing the model.

The interviews with nurse managers measured their work experience, level of management training, and leadership style, because these variables would be expected to influence staff nurses' work satisfaction and retention. Although PPM nurse managers had approximately 4 more years of nursing work experience than managers of traditional units, there were no differences in amount of management experience. Leadership style, including measures of task and relationship dimensions of leader behavior, did not differ significantly between the two groups of nurse managers. We conclude that the small sample size (eight nurse managers in each group) was not sufficient to detect differences in leadership style between the two groups of head nurses.

With regard to effects of the PPM on patients, findings were mixed (Cassard, Weisman, Gordon, & Wong, in press). In comparisons of patients discharged from PPM units with patients discharged from matched TM units, no effects of the PPM on patient satisfaction with nursing care, or with overall hospital care, could be found. The only significant difference between the two groups of patients on day of discharge was that patients discharged from PPM units were more likely to be able to name their primary nurse. The conclusion, therefore, is that the PPM has no effect, either positive or negative, on patient satisfaction with care received.

The analysis of patient outcomes revealed, at the bivariate level, no significant differences between the two groups of patients on perceived health or functional status, on unplanned health care utilization, or on hospital readmission. Bivariate analyses of needs and unmet needs 2 weeks post discharge revealed significantly more treatment-related needs and needs related to activities of daily living (ADLs) and instrumental ADLs among patients discharged from PPM units. This occurred, in part, because patients with musculoskeletal diagnoses tended to report more needs, and these patients were treated almost exclusively on PPM units. (Randomizing patients with similar diagnoses to PPM or traditional units would have improved the design of the study for assessing patient outcomes, but this was not possible at JHH.) Controlling for patient and hospitalization characteristics in multivariate analyses revealed no significant effects, either positive or negative, of the PPM on postdischarge unmet needs for care.

The overall conclusion from the patient outcome component of the evaluation is that the PPM has no discernible impact, either positive or negative, on patient outcomes. Hence the PPM can be said to maintain the quality of patient care while improving nurses' work satisfaction and retention. One possible explanation for the null findings with regard to effects on patient outcomes is that any group synergies expected based on the theory of self-managed work groups might have been offset by the tendency of nurses on the PPM units to maximize their chances of receiving gain-sharing payoffs by, for example, working longer hours or keeping permanent nurse staffing levels low. The latter would be consistent with a utility maximization view of human behavior, given the gain-sharing incentive, and might be expected to have negative effects on patient care.

Finally, with regard to unit costs, expenditures for nursing staff were compared for PPM and TM units for calendar year 1990, using data from hospital records. Operating rooms (ORs) and inpatient units were compared separately. To compare costs adjusted by output across units, ratios of dollars for nursing personnel per patient day were used for inpatient units, and dollars for nursing personnel per amount of time of operating room use were used for ORs. For inpatient units, results show that the cost per patient day is slightly lower on

PPM units than on traditional units, although the difference is not significant. For ORs, the cost per OR day is significantly higher on PPM units as compared with traditional units.

These results can be traced in part to the different mix of nursing personnel used. PPM inpatient units used fewer purchased nursing services and nursing aides than traditional units, but PPM inpatient units employed similar numbers of RNs at upgraded salaries; the result is similar nursing costs. PPM ORs, however, used more hours of RN time, resulting in overall higher nursing costs.

Several limitations of the cost analysis should be noted. First, trend data in unit costs have not yet been analyzed. Second, the analysis omits an important source of hospital nursing costs, the cost of recruitment and orientation of new nursing staff, that could only be estimated for 1 year for the study units. Although the estimates reveal higher costs for recruitment and orientation for TM units than for PPM units, the differences are not significant.

The conclusion from the cost analyses conducted so far is that there does not appear to be an overall cost savings attributable to the PPM. However, it is clear that the PPM encourages less use of purchased nursing services and of nursing aides. It may also encourage more intensive use of RNs in ORs.

The overall conclusion of the evaluation study is that the PPM accomplishes the objectives it was originally designed to achieve, namely, improving the work satisfaction and retention levels of nurses. With regard to other outcomes, the PPM was found to maintain the quality of patient care, as evidenced by no effects, either positive or negative, on patient satisfaction levels or on post-discharge patient outcomes. The PPM also was found to have no impact on unit costs for inpatient units (because reductions in costs for purchased nursing services are offset by higher costs for RNs), but to increase the unit costs for ORs.

DISCUSSION

Contemporary nurse executives seek empirical data in order to make informed decisions about alternative models of nursing care delivery. This study is important because it provides information on three areas of outcomes of the redesign of nurses' work in several clinical areas, permitting the executive to consider more than one aspect of its effectiveness. The unit self-management model at JHH was evaluated for its effect on nurses, patients, and costs. The study's other contribution is the conceptualization and measurement of the links between the model components and outcomes, which are essential steps in efforts to improve both the quality and efficiency of patient care in contemporary organizations.

The PPM was found to be associated with nurses' higher work satisfaction and retention. Higher work satisfaction was due, in part, to the PPM's improvement of two aspects of work process: teamwork and coordination of care. These findings provide useful information regarding self-managed work groups theory because these variables correspond to Hackman's observations of group synergy and efficiency in work process.

Because the PPM was in part designed to increase nurses' control over decision making and the work schedules of the unit, an unanticipated finding was that nurses' perceptions of their autonomy did not predict work satisfaction. Autonomy has been the most frequent variable cited in previous work satisfaction studies (Blegen, 1993). Its failure to predict satisfaction here may reflect the changing context of care or the possibility that nurse participation in decision making has actually improved over time. Another consideration is that primary nursing, which enhances autonomy, has been in practice at JHH for over a decade. In such settings, the nurse manager may want to consider emphasizing work processes of groups in building management models, rather than autonomy.

Such strategies would be consistent with today's emphasis on continuous quality improvement (CQI). According to Dienemann (1992), "CQI is a process that assumes that work groups are experts about their work and should be the focus for monitoring quality, identifying problems and devising solutions" (p. 27). The use of professional teams in the process of identifying, monitoring, and evaluating quality requires developing skills relevant to work processes. PPM nurses, as expected, spend more time in unit management activities. For the nurse executive, however, it is important to note that this did not take away from direct or indirect patient care hours.

As reported, there were contrasting findings related to retention and satisfaction: Longer hours reported by PPM nurses are associated with decreased satisfaction, and PPM nurses receive higher pay, which leads to increased retention. The nurse executive considering implementation of self-managed units would need to weigh this information carefully.

Another conclusion from this study is that the PPM maintains the quality of patient care. This suggests that nurse executives who desire models of care that facilitate improvement of patient care outcomes must weigh the value of being able to maintain patient care in relation to changes that improve nurse satisfaction and retention.

Whether new nursing care delivery models raise or lower costs in the hospital setting in relation to the more traditional approaches is a question of concern (Gardner & Tilbury, 1991). The PPM inpatient units had costs similar to those of TM units. However, nurse executives may need to consider differences in types of units when implementing compensation strategies, in light of the finding that ORs had greater costs attributable to more registered nurse time.

SUMMARY

The PPM is a redesign of nurses' work and was derived from organization, human relations, and nursing concepts. Intended primarily to decrease sources of dissatisfaction and increase retention at the time of its inception (1980), there were expectations that patient care would be improved and that decreased utilization of temporary personnel would reduce costs. This recent evaluation (1990) of the effects of the PPM at JHH on nurses, patients, and costs revealed that the model appears to be working. Professional practice units have higher satisfaction and higher retention, maintain quality of patient care, and are cost-neutral on inpatient units. At the time of the investigation, the PPM had diffused to 16 hospital units, none of which had ever returned to traditional unit management.

The PPM is consistent with contemporary philosophy and principles of continuous quality improvement, which include decentralization of quality monitoring and evaluation, and the use of nursing and interdisciplinary teams. Other hospitals have adopted the PPM as described here, and differing aspects of nursing self-management are employed elsewhere. Studies to evaluate the effectiveness of such reorganization of nursing resources beyond the one setting described would help determine its suitability and transferability to other settings and further test the theoretical and conceptual models employed.

REFERENCES

Alexander, C. S., Weisman, C. S., & Chase, G. A. (1981). Evaluating primary nursing in hospitals: Examinations of effects on nursing staff. *Medical Care, 19,* 80-89.

Blegen, M. A. (1993). Nurses' job satisfaction: A meta-analysis of related variables. *Nursing Research, 42*(1), 36-41.

Cassard, S. D., Weisman, C. S., Gordon, D. L., & Wong, R. (in press). The impact of unit-based self management by nurses on patient outcomes. *Health Services Research.*

Dear, M. R., Weisman, C. S., & O'Keefe, S. (1985). Evaluation of a contract model for professional nursing practice. *Health Care Management Review, 10*(2), 65-77.

Dienemann, J. (1992). Approaches to quality improvement. In J. Dienemann (Ed.), *Continuous quality improvement in nursing* (p. 27). Washington, DC: American Nurses Association.

Friss, L. (1982). Hospital nurse staffing: An urgent need for management reappraisal. *Health Care Management, 7*(1), 21-27.

Gardner, K. G., & Tilbury, M. (1991). A longitudinal cost analysis of primary and team nursing. Nursing Economics, 9(2), 97-104.

Goodman, P. S., Davadas, R., & Hughson, T. L. (1988). Groups and productivity: Analyzing the effectiveness of self-managing teams. In J. P. Campbell & R. J. Campbell (Eds.), *Productivity in organizations: New perspectives from organizational and industrial psychology* (pp. 275-327). San Francisco: Jossey-Bass.

Hackman, J. R. (1990). Work teams in organizations: An orienting framework. In J. R. Hackman (Ed.), *Groups that work (and those that don't)* (pp. 1-14). San Francisco: Jossey-Bass.

Hackman, J. R., & Lawler, E. E. (1971). Employee reactions to job characteristics. *Journal of Applied Psychology, 55,* 259-286.

Hackman, J. R., & Oldham, G. R. (1976). Motivation through the design of work: Test of a theory. *Organizational Behavior and Human Performance, 16,* 250-279.

Hackman, J. R., & Oldham, G. R. (1980). *Work redesign.* Reading, MA: Addison-Wesley.

Kramer, M. (1974). *Reality shock: Why nurses leave nursing.* St. Louis: C. V. Mosby.

Price, J. L., & Mueller, C. W. (1981). *Professional turnover: The case of nurses.* New York: Spectrum.

Rose, M., & DiPasquale, B. (1990). The Johns Hopkins professional practice model. In G. G. Mayer, M. J. Madden, & E. Fawreng (Eds.), *Patient care delivery models* (pp. 85-97). Rockville, MD: Aspen.

Sethi, A. S., Berkwood, P. L., & Schuler, R. S. (1989). The role of job design and job analysis in the strategic human resource management mode. In A. S. Sethi & R. S. Shuler (Eds.), *Human resource management in the health care sector* (pp. 41-73). New York: Quorum.

U.S. Department of Health and Human Services. (1988). *Secretary's Commission on Nursing* (Final Report, Vol. 1). Washington, DC: U.S. Government Printing Office.

Weisman, C. S. (1982). Recruit from within: Hospital nurse retention in 1980's. *Journal of Nursing Administration, 12,* 24-31.

Weisman, C. S. (1991, September). *Nursing practice models: Research on patient outcomes.* Paper presented at the National Conference for Nursing Research on Patient Outcomes Research: The Effectiveness of Nursing Practice, Bethesda, MD.

Weisman, C. S., Alexander, C. S., & Chase, G. A. (1981). Determinants of hospital staff nurse turnover. *Medical Care, 19,* 431.

Weisman, C. S., Gordon, D. L., Cassard, S. D., Bergner, M., & Wong, R. (1993). The effects of unit self management on hospital nurses' work process, work satisfaction, and retention. *Medical Care, 31,* 318-393.

CHAPTER 15

Successful and "Failed" Work Redesign Projects: Illuminating the Creative Tension

Carolyn L. Brown

The spirit of work redesign, according to Hackman and Oldham (1980), encompasses planning for work that is both productive and fun. This chapter (a) explores the spirit of work redesign in nursing, (b) provides a thematic analysis of successful work redesign processes reported in the literature, and (c) describes the creative tension (Senge, 1991) within "failed" work redesign. On the basis of the illumination of gaps in the existing literature and the creative tension existing in "failed" projects, suggestions are offered for engaging in work redesign with recognition that organizational conditions may be less than optimal.

"Lots of jobs are not so well designed. They demotivate people rather than turn them on. They undermine rather than encourage productivity and work quality. They aren't any fun" (Hackman & Oldham, 1980, p. ix). The work done by nurses in most of today's health care delivery systems still fits this description of unfulfilling work. In fact, work for most nurses has not changed substantively during this century. Technology and knowledge of nursing have both exploded since the 1940s, but there have been no meaningful changes in the way nursing work is constructed. Generally, nurses still work in hospitals in basically task-oriented systems. Nurses come out of nursing schools feeling enthusiastic about nursing work, only to find, after a year of practice in most acute care settings, that they feel highly stressed and wish to find a job outside of acute care, and sometimes outside of nursing.

Since the mid-1980's and in response to the latest nursing shortage, nurses have been engaged in efforts to discern the causes for disenchantment with nursing work. In order to stem the tide of nurses leaving acute care settings or leaving nursing altogether, and to meet the mandates of economic restraints, leaders in nursing have initiated nursing work redesign efforts. In fact, *work redesign* is the latest buzzword in health care organizations and nursing. Leaders in nursing and the health care industry see it as the way we will save ourselves, our institutions, and our clients, and elevate nursing practice. Yet much of the literature on work redesign and recent experiences of the author in work settings elicit a sense of déjà vu—a sense that what is being seen is all too familiar. In an effort to find a quick fix that is palatable to all, persons in leadership positions seem to be trying to solve the same old problems by using the same old solutions, or by trying radically new solutions doomed to fail because they are embedded in the same old structures.

THE SPIRIT OF WORK REDESIGN IN NURSING

Hackman and Oldham (1980) believed that "jobs can be set up so that work and fun are not so often at opposite poles of people's experiences, and so that productivity does not have to be at the expense of the satisfaction and growth of the people who do the producing" (p. x). The only references to fun in literature on nursing work was found in McCloskey's (1991) guest editorial, which speaks of the need to include " 'big fun'—the good feeling we get from being creative, making others feel good, and being good at what we do"—in nursing work (p. 5). Similar to this view of fun is Simms' notion of work excitement, defined as the sense of "personal enthusiasm and commitment for work evidenced by creativity, receptivity to learning, and ability to see opportunity in everyday situations" (Simms, Erbin-Roesemann, Darga, & Coeling, 1990, p. 178).

So at the heart of work redesign is the notion of fun, excitement, enthusiasm, and energy generated from work. All of these are concepts much fuller than the idea of work satisfaction, a variable often used to determine how well jobs are constructed. Work satisfaction implies that "things are O.K.," that people are content and pleased, but excitement, exhilaration, energy, and joy in creating are not included. In fact, satisfaction speaks to a certain level of adaptation. As Hackman and Oldham (1980) noted, adapting often occurs in work situations in which people do not believe they can have an impact on creating a better situation for themselves or others. In most nursing work situations, nurses have learned to adapt: to put in their eight-plus hours, put up with the conditions, do as they are told, gather their checks, and go home. They have not been asked to contribute to the organization in a creative way. In fact, many nurses have experienced negative consequences for suggesting that things might be done differently. So adaptation and acquiescence become the way to survive. When work becomes too unhappy, nurses express their displeasure by moving on to a different work situation in which there is hope that things might be different. Thus the attempt to cope with poor work situations becomes a search for an external utopian solution to the day-to-day struggle with nursing work—and the turnover/retention issue that surfaces over and over again in the literature as nurses struggle to find meaningful ways to express their art (Pierce, Freund, Luikart, & Fondren, 1991; Prescott, 1986; Robinson et al., 1991; Wise, 1993). When enough nurses have become disenchanted and enough work situations are nonresponsive, we have another nursing shortage.

Over 13 years ago, Hackman and Oldham (1980) highlighted the need for actual restructuring of the work that people do to move it away from the machinelike orientation of typical factory and bureaucratic jobs. Their call was for radically new ways of envisioning work. Non-health-care industries heeded this call, and new structures emerged. Saturn, a division of General Motors, is a good example (Sanford & Mang, 1993, p. 159). Yet nursing work has not fared so well. Kerfoot (1988) states,

> The research consistently tells us that nurses leave hospital nursing because they do not feel a sense of autonomy, control over their practice, or respect as a professional. They do not have sufficient input into the system. Although these needs could easily be addressed through a professional model of nursing, hospitals have been reluctant to do so. (p. 321)

Many of the books and articles on work redesign projects in nursing smack of the same old refrain. Most, in fact, seem to apply new language to old solutions to old problems by using words like *primary nursing, partners in practice,* and *case management* to describe systems that are basically team nursing. Without the philosophical shift and appropriate supports, the structure of work stays the same. What is missing is a focus on the values and principles undergirding the concepts (Manthey, 1992). Rather than creating system-level changes that tackle the underlying assumptions, enthusiastic executives embrace a new care delivery model in form and name, but do not do the necessary homework to make the change viable in their organizations.

Neither the organization nor the people in the organizations are ready to embrace the change and make it theirs. The solution becomes a band-aid approach with little chance to succeed in a basically hostile environment. An analogy is doing a kidney transplant, using a stranger's kidney, without learning whether the body systems are compatible and without working to suppress the immune system of the recipient. Solutions in name only will not create meaningful changes in nursing work. In fact, when speaking of changes that tend to be at the level of language rather than substantive organizational change, Manthey (1992) stated, "It is disrespectful to use language so carelessly. The energy we waste dealing with dilution and distortions of our finest innovations would be better spent developing true creativity for future challenges" (p. 21).

The spirit of work redesign, in the tradition of Hackman and Oldham (1980), is to restructure work for productivity *and* fun for those doing the work. Nurses and others in health care systems have grabbed onto the *productivity* part as if it were a life raft for floundering systems, but have not done so well with the *fun* part.

THE PROCESS OF SUCCESSFUL WORK REDESIGN: WHAT ARE THE THEMES?

In searching the nursing literature for successful work redesign projects, the author found few actual descriptions of the process of projects. There were many conceptual, editorial, and research articles, but few descriptions of the way a project unfolded. Process data were chosen to elicit themes leading to successful work redesign projects because those initiating work redesign efforts need to know what has potential for creating a successful venture. Although it would have been helpful to know what did not work well, this type of information was absent in the literature.

Descriptions of the process of nursing work redesign were found in the Nursing Administration Quarterly section labeled "On the Scene" ("On the Scene: Executive Teamwork," 1989; "On the Scene: Hoag," 1991; "On the Scene: Managed Care," 1993; "On the Scene: Nurse Empowerment," 1992; "On the Scene: On the Move," 1991; "On the Scene: Restructuring," 1991; "On the Scene: Section I," 1987, 1990; "On the Scene: Section II," 1987). These sections described ongoing efforts within nursing organizations to redesign nursing work. The sections were long and differed widely as to content, but did, in fact, provide the most useful data about what might make a work redesign project successful. Though used as data for thematic analysis, the reports were intended

TABLE 15.1   Selected Successful Work Redesign Project Descriptions

Project	Source	Number Reporting
Riverview Medical Center—Positive environment for professional practice	"On the Scene: Section I," 1987	20
Riverview Medical Center—Nurse empowerment	"On the Scene: Nurse Empowerment," 1992	22
Beth Israel Hospital—Geronotological Nursing Program	"On the Scene: Section I," 1990; Clifford & Horvath, 1990	8
Beth Israel Hospital—Advancing Professional Nursing Practice	"On the Scene: Section I," 1990; Clifford & Horvath, 1990	28
University of California-San Francisco—Decentralization and participation	"On the Scene: Section II," 1987	6
John's Hopkins Hospital—Managed care	"On the Scene: Managed care," 1993	8
Hoag Memorial Hospital—Product Line	"On the Scene: Hoag Memorial," 1991	3
Michigan Medical Center—Executive teamwork	"On the Scene: Executive Teamwork," 1989	6
Mercy Health Services—Restructuring nursing	"On the Scene: Restructuring," 1991	11
Tallahassee Memorial Regional Medical Center and Mercy Health Services Nursing Council—Interactive planning	"On the Scene: Restructuring," 1991	48

to be only descriptions of successful projects. Clifford and Horvath's (1990) book on Beth Israel's experience with work redesign was also included.

Table 15.1 is a list of the projects selected for inclusion in the thematic analysis of successful projects. This list is by no means comprehensive, reflecting simply the literature that (a) emerged from the literature search, (b) was a process description of a work redesign effort, and (c) was available to the author.

Analyzing any data for themes is a complex process. It involves reading and rereading data for commonalities to make sense of the "mess" of data. "Theme gives shape to the shapeless . . . describes the content . . . [and] is always a reduction of a notion" (van Manen, 1990, p. 88). Themes, rather than categories, were chosen to illuminate the commonalities among the projects because the descriptions yielded overlapping meaning structures rather than crisp exclusive categories.

It Takes a Diverse Group

One of the most significant themes noted was that descriptions were written by groups of persons who had participated in the project. For example, Beth Israel's story was told by 28 people (Clifford & Horvath, 1990), Riverview Medical Center's, under the leadership of Joan Trofino, was told by 22 persons, and the report on interactive planning at Tallahassee Memorial Regional Medical Center and Mercy Health Services ("On the Scene—Restructuring," 1991) was told by two groups totaling 48 in number. Who the storytellers were indicates the levels and complexity of participation necessary for successful systems-level work redesign projects. Thus the first, and overriding, theme that emerged from descriptions was the necessity for widespread participation at all levels of the planning and implementation processes of successful nursing work redesign.

Successful work redesign projects come from the vision of many, with leaders acting as coordinators and facilitators. Embedded in this theme is the commitment of participants to the values undergirding the project and the worth of the project itself. The number and types of participants indicate the need for diverse persons and perspectives in the planning process. Participants in successful projects were from many levels in the organizations, represented a wide diversity of educational backgrounds and positions, and often included disciplines other than nursing. The diversity of persons participating in work redesign projects is in keeping with strategies that will serve nursing well as we move into organizing for the future. Newer thinking in business demonstrates a trend toward systems thinking and breaking down the strong departmental and professional boundaries. Indicative of this trend in health care planning is the formation of multidisciplinary quality improvement teams to better serve clients. Nursing can rarely afford to plan alone, whether on a unit or organization-wide level.

It Takes Time

Another dominant theme was that successful work redesign takes time. Projects ranged from smaller pilot activities to organization-wide activities to multiorganization systemwide change. Some began on a smaller level and moved to organization-wide change. Others began at the larger organization or system level. Of particular interest was the Riverview Project, which was reported in 1987 and again in 1992, with a consistent theme of creating an environment to empower nurses to practice as professionals. One can see the growth in the project since its inception. Beth Israel's story began in 1973 and is ongoing. Clifford and Horvath (1990), also with a focus on creating a professional practice environment, observed that Beth Israel contracted to tell their story through the medium of a book over a decade ago, but found themselves unable to do so until 1990 because "simply, it takes time for change to become an integral part of an organizations's culture and the development of a professional practice system at Beth Israel Hospital was no exception" (p. 300). Systems-level projects unfolded in a time frame of years.

It Lacks Research

A major gap in descriptions of projects is due to the newness and messiness of the endeavors. Often a project is not undertaken with the idea of systematic tracking of process in mind. With one exception (Mercy Health Services Consortium), no projects reported a research method to manage and analyze data. Mercy's consortium reported using "two approaches to analysis: (1) a naturalistic methodology for analysis of the transcribed data, and (2) a traditional content analysis of the flip-chart data" (Porter, 1991, p. 46) generated during planning. Though initial assessment and ongoing evaluation were often built into the projects, reports of projects tended to be retrospective recall of process without systematic presentation of data used to track the process. While engaged in the process, people tend to be aware of what does and does not work, but in the day-to-day world of practice and of responding to immediate needs, the stories of success need to be reconstructed from memory, minutes, and other documents. Testimony to this fact is this statement: "Few, if any, of the solutions to 'restructuring for change' models or plans have been field tested for any length of time. Research findings are simply not available" (Beyers, 1991, p. 44).

It Takes Participation

Participation was another theme that consistently appeared in the descriptions and emerged from the project descriptions in several different contexts. For example, participation was uniformly described as a part of the planning process for a project. People in organizations were asked to participate in a number of ways. In many cases, broad input about the status of an organization was sought as part of creating baseline data from which to begin the change process. This was the most elementary level of participation—providing input for others to make decisions. Participation also appeared in the sense of persons' being an integral part of the change process through membership on a planning team or engaging in ongoing decisions relative to implementing a project on a unit. Participation was often a goal of planning processes: For example, an aim of a project might be more meaningful participation for employees. This goal was sometimes expressed through the setting up of shared governance structures.

Another way participation emerged as a theme from the descriptions of projects was through decentralizing authority, accountability, and responsibility to the lowest level possible in the organization. When participation is most effective, there is a conscious effort by the leadership to relinquish control. "Most important is the willingness to share power with all nurses in an organization, thus empowering them to succeed and achieve personal and organizational goals and finally to help create a more powerful total nursing organization for all" (Trofino, 1987, p. 11). Trofino went on to state that the ultimate in creating empowered participation in the work of nursing organizations is "recognizing nurses' expertise, trusting them, and sharing power with them. The primary role of leaders will be to empower others to be their own leaders" (Trofino, 1992, p. 23). When projects were successful, the participation of many went into planning, implementing, and maintaining the project.

It Requires Diagnostic Data

Hackman and Oldham (1980) described the next theme. They emphasized the importance of "collecting diagnostic data about a work system before it is redesigned" (p. xi). This allows work redesign project participants to tailor changes to their own unique systems. Most successful redesign projects gathered data about the existing system before they engaged in implementing change. As previously noted, the degree of systematization and level of sophistication of the data management process varied widely.

It Has a Systems Perspective

Most of the projects reported some level of systems orientation. This varied from a recognition of the interactive and integrated nature of creating change to recognizing the needs of the community of persons served as an extension of the system. Systems thinking is awareness of the interconnection of the whole. What happens in one part of a system affects the whole system. One important way systems thinking was expressed was in the approach to redesigning systems. Most projects involved more than nursing. *Collaboration* was a word that surfaced repeatedly in relation to different levels of the organization, physicians and nursing, nursing and other professionals, other departments, and across organizations in multiorganization systems. *Collaboration* meant egalitarian participation in the redesign process by the collaborators. Part of systems thinking is viewing service in relation to populations rather than individuals. One project participant reported, "I can identify more clearly the patient population with whom I am most involved" ("On the Scene: Section I," 1990, p. 14). Similarly, "At Hoag Memorial Hospital, head nurses have access to annual community survey data so they are able to evaluate shifts in demographics, predict changes, and suggest modifications to product lines in order to remain competitive" (Vosburgh, 1991, pp. 42-43).

It Starts With Values

Another theme, although not predominant in the projects, is the notion of starting the project with a basic philosophical assessment highlighting the values and assumptions undergirding the redesign process. Rabkin (1990), a physician and the president of Beth Israel Medical Center, stated, "The rationale [for Beth Israel's redesign project] is straightforward, the hospital is fundamentally a nursing institution and not one of doctoring" (1990, p. 7). This statement highlights the central position of nursing in the redesign process. The primary concept in Beth Israel's Professional Nursing Practice Model (PNPM) is "the caring relationship between the patient/family and the nurse. Thus the focus of the PNPM and the fulcrum on which all other concepts of the Model are balanced is the construct of Patient/Family-Nurse Interrelationship" (Rempusheski, 1990, pp. 286-287). The rest of the model, planning, and redesign flowed from this basic premise adopted by the system.

Other projects began with assumptions and values about nurses as professional practitioners—for example, "the nurse as a knowledge specialist" ("On the Scene: Nurse Empowerment," 1990, p. 22). For nurses to be considered knowledge specialists, knowledge development becomes a critical component of work redesign. Joan Trofino spoke of enacting this philosophy: "Educational commitment is essential in an empowered nursing organization. . . . A nurse executive who is a perpetual learner will create an environment where staff education is expected, rewarded and valued. All educational programs should be available to any interested nurses regardless of content" ("On the Scene: Nurse Empowerment," 1990, p. 21). In several projects, knowledge was seen as undergirding clinical expertise and as a requisite for engaging actively in professionalizing nursing work.

It Takes Education

The need for ongoing education was another theme present in successful work redesign projects. Work redesign created a demand for preparation to meet the expectations of new role expectations for all participants. Hackman and Oldham (1980) noted that people adapt to what exists. Knowledge and skills that were effective in helping people adapt to existing systems do not necessarily work well in redesigned systems. Education occurred on many levels throughout the reviewed projects. Orientation sessions were necessary for key players in planning processes. Educational programs assisted people to gain knowledge for enacting expanded roles. Educational programs were set in place to orient newcomers to the new systems in order to maintain system integrity. Where appropriate, clients were educated to become effective participants in planning systems of care for populations and for themselves.

"FAILED" WORK REDESIGN PROJECTS

The previous section described themes characterizing successful work redesign projects. In all cases, projects described processes that worked, that culminated in desired outcomes. When surveying the literature on work redesign, one wonders what happens to those projects labeled "unsuccessful," or even more bluntly, projects that "failed." It is as though all "failures" drop into a "black hole," disappearing forever. Much can be learned from projects that do not succeed in the traditional sense, that fail to meet their objectives as conceptualized at the beginning.

The author has been a part of a number of work redesign efforts in a number of roles over the span of her career: manager of a nursing unit, researcher, consultant, and participant observer. Some of the projects have been successful and some not. In two cases, the projects were aborted and might, in a traditional sense, be termed "failures." Certainly, the original objectives for the projects were not met. In both cases, the projects involved participatory action research perspectives with a high degree of participation on the parts of persons within the system. In one, data were gathered by a department in the organization about the existing organization and were analyzed for common themes. The overarching theme was a desire for more meaningful participation by persons working in the system. Specific recommendations for action to achieve greater participation at all levels of the organization were crafted and submitted through appropriate channels. At this point, the project floundered. The second "failed" project again involved a department in a larger organization. In this project the department developed a strategic plan for redesign and began to craft a plan to gather data about the department and the organization in a systematic way. Several groups had been involved with planning ways to further develop and implement a strategic plan agreed upon by the nursing management group at a full-day retreat. At the point of having agreed to the data-gathering method and instrumentation, and being poised to start, the project floundered. Neither project was resurrected, and after anger and dismay at the outcomes, the organizations involved continued operations, with the projects having made little impact.

Both of these projects were started in good faith but were probably doomed to fail from the outset. In both cases, the projects were started by a department, and although part of the planning had been to ascertain who needed to be involved in the planning, either the assessment was faulty or the permissions given did not demonstrate full support for the projects. Hackman and Oldham (1980) recommended a full assessment of the organization prior to beginning to redesign work. They spoke of diagnosing the system: "Even if we knew precisely what it was about a given job that most required improvement, it would be foolhardy to start making those changes without some indication of the *readiness of the people for change* and the *hospitality of the organization* to getting the changes installed" (Hackman & Oldham, 1980, p. 117).

Underlying the issues of readiness of people for change and hospitality of the organization is the matter of expectations grounded in different world-views. Senge (1991) noted that most of our primary institutions in this country are geared toward controlling rather than creating. Organizations are generally founded on the idea that "the name of the game is getting the right answer and avoiding mistakes" (p. 89). Leaders in typical traditional health care organizations also operate according to this premise. Thus to gather data about the realities of an organization may well strike fear into the hearts of leaders in organizations in which perfection in the form of needing to be right, coupled with low to no tolerance for mistakes, exists as an underlying value. Adding insult to injury was the fact that the impetus for change came from a department rather than from the top leadership. This assault on tradition was particularly damaging because it struck to the core of assumptions and beliefs about the nature of work and workers. Tradition has leaders cast in the role of "special people who set the direction, make the key decisions, and energize the troops.... [This view] is deeply rooted in an individualistic and non-systematic worldview" (Senge, 1991, p. 91). In such organizations, the norm is keeping things as they are. In traditional organizations there is no knowledge or tolerance for the notion of "creative tension. Creative tension comes from seeing clearly where we want to be, our 'vision,' and telling the truth about where we are, our 'current reality' " (Senge, 1991, p. 92).

People in organizations create beautiful, nicely bound and labeled notebooks full of wonderful visionary plans for the future, and these plans gather dust on the shelves because there is no desire to look at the tension between the current reality and the wonderful vision. Wheatley (1992) likened most of today's organizations to "impressive fortresses" (p. 16) permeated by defensive language and ways of interacting. They are characterized by chains of command that control who talks to whom about what. Fear motivates people to engage in protective ways of being and interacting. Lack of trust in one another's competence and motivation is common. Efforts to create change by people in lower echelons are taken to be slurs on the competence of managers, and thus have little chance to succeed. A lot of effort goes into underground communication systems in which the talk is about the enemy or "them."

The fundamental values undergirding genuine participation had not yet permeated the organizations in which efforts to redesign work "failed." Nor had the idea that engaging in change processes affects the whole system. Systems thinking was nonexistent. Another reason for the demise of these projects was the failure to assess the impact of change on the rest of the organization. In both cases, the decision-making rules would have changed within the departments redesigning work, resulting in new demands on the rest of the organization. In neither project were other departments invited to participate, probably generating fear of the unknown for nonparticipants.

In today's health care environment, nursing is most often practiced within health care organizations. Most of these organizations struggle to survive, let alone engage in creative redesign. Land and Jarman (1993) spoke to the notion of breakpoint changes that occur when the organization moves to a radically different phase in its development. They described three points in an organization's development when breakpoint change occurs: (a) organizational start-up, when entrepreneurship is demanded, (b) movement to stabilizing for efficient system maintenance, and (c) movement from maintenance to reinvention to survive. The third breakpoint change is most difficult because it involves a "cycle of rebirth" requiring significant changes in internal controls and a sense of creative energy. This is where health care organizations are now, like dinosaurs waiting for the coming changes in the health care system. What are needed at this breakpoint are two types of change: innovation and invention. Neither is welcomed by the dinosaur. Instead, most organizations fall back on what has worked in the past. Control is centralized, micromanagement prevails, the workforce is cut in order to survive economically, and workers are pushed to the wall to produce more for less. Just when control needs to be less, it becomes more. When the organization needs to be most flexible, it becomes most rigid. The meaning of work becomes even more machinelike and grueling, rather than exciting and fun. Certainly, efforts by the workers in organizations to make work more meaningful take a second seat to the bottom line. People are so busy responding that there is no time to create. So, as described by Hackman and Oldham (1980), we have workers, in this case nurses, adapting to sick, energy-draining systems.

Had the redesign planners in either of these two departments done an adequate job of assessing their organizations, these two projects might never have been started. In neither case were the organizations friendly to change. In one, the hospital had existed in the community for over 25 years and had succeeded by operating much like the hospitals described by Ashley (1976) in *Hospitals, Paternalism, and the Role of the Nurse*. The chief executive officer was Papa and the director of Nursing was Mama, with the rest of the organization filling out the family roles. When new players moved into these roles, the rest of the organization did not change, and in fact many of the characteristics of these two roles remained the same. Informal organizational norms crafted these roles. Control of the organization was highly centralized, with the CEO in the position of final authority. In addition, there was tension, divisiveness, and mistrust within the department itself. Despite the best of intentions and a high degree of need for redesigned work, the organization was not ready to undertake substantive redesign work. In organizations that are mired in the struggle to maintain themselves in the old ways of doing things, there is no creative tension between what is and what is envisioned. Visionary and hopeful plans can be made by those trapped in jobs designed to preserve the status quo. However, if leaders in the organization have little desire to examine data about the current state of the organization and are unwilling to see with a new lens, little change is possible. Those who are not in top leadership roles and who desire change also need to look at the whole with the same willingness to assess what exists in relation to what is hoped for. Recognition of the readiness of the total organization to engage in redesign is a part of this process. When change in nursing work is so desperately needed, nurses are tempted to look through the rosy lens of hope, rather than the clear lens geared to "see it like it is." The starting point for the creative tension necessary for change is the gap between the vision and the present reality. When there is little organizational support for a redesign project, abandoning system-level redesign efforts in order to first work to create an environment more friendly to redesign efforts may be a wise plan.

SUGGESTIONS FOR REENVISIONING CHANGE PROCESSES

This section presents some unconventional ways to respond to the change process. Some may be especially meaningful for those caught within dinosaur organizations fearful of change.

Starting With the Self

"No problem can be solved from the same consciousness that created it. We must learn to see the world anew" (Wheatley, 1992, p. 5). Leaders in nursing are caught up in the same mind traps as the rest of the people in dinosaur health care organizations. Nurse leaders would do well to start with intensive introspective work in order to reveal the assumptions that guide their beliefs about nursing work and the ways that work is organized. What do you truly believe about nursing work, not at the level of what you are expected to believe, but at the gut level of action? Your deeply held assumptions and values are expressed in your day-to-day decisions and actions. What do your actions tell you about what you believe and value? Though not spoken of in the literature on planning work redesign projects, starting with the self is a necessary first step. Other questions to ask yourself might be: How patient am I? How willing am I to see the unpleasant truths about myself and my own department? How willing am I to see the truth about organizational realities, and to start the process where it needs to start for this organization? Do I trust the good will, motivations, and competencies of my coworkers—on the executive team, in my department/ division, of other departments, of the chief executive officer? Given that trust is not global, what do I trust them for? How much control do I maintain? How willing and able am I to let go of control and allow genuine full participation? A good question to ask yourself is, How well do I think this department and this organization could function without me? Does my honest answer to this question threaten me? Answers to questions like these will inform decisions about how to proceed with work redesign. The place to begin work redesign is within the self with a serious appraisal of one's own beliefs, assumptions, and values related to nursing work and the organizations in which that work occurs. This reflective work should be ongoing and honest.

Learning About the Meaning
of Nursing Work in the Organization

With other people, explore the focus of nursing work. In redesigning nursing work, engaging in conversations with others to learn their worldview assumptions about work, and in particular, nursing work, is part of the foundational preparation that needs to occur. Ask questions such as: What makes work meaningful for you? How does work fit into creating a meaningful life? Do you believe work should promote health and well-being? What should be the primary objective of work? Rosen (1991) also proposed searching for the assumptions that undergird an organization. He stated, "Healthy companies all possess and emanate a certain vitality and spirit . . . a deep feeling of shared humanistic values at the core of the company. . . . They circulate through every cell and artery of the company, and a company and its employees either reinforce healthy values or bring about their decline" (Rosen, 1991, p. 123). Leaders committed to creating healthy companies recognize that "work can either make people sick or improve their health. The physical and psychological climate at work plays an enormous role in well-being and performance"

(Rosen, 1991, p. 126). When healthy work situations are at the heart of work redesign, productivity follows. Healthy work situations do not start with stress reduction programs. Instead they begin with finding the source of stress to create work with healthy rather than illness-producing levels of tension. If caring is found to be the essence of nursing work, then nurses need to extend that value to their own populations in the sense of creating health-promoting work.

What populations do we serve? Traditionally, we look at client populations. For example, Packard, Schultz, and Graham (1993) proposed redesigning curriculum for nursing administration around a population focus. One group rarely considered as a recipient of care is the population of nurses. In redesigning nursing work, many of the projects reviewed for this chapter started from knowing that something was wrong with the way nursing work is organized. None of them spoke about the well-being of the nurse as a focus for work redesign. One population desperately in need of health promoting work redesign is nurses. Another is other staff who work in health care organizations. Work redesign can promote healing for individuals and organizations for health care providers and recipients.

Finding Alternatives to System-Level Work Redesign

Nurses can engage in work redesign efforts on many different levels. Many of the successful redesign projects started as pilot projects, or began with a small segment of the organization. Perhaps starting with one's own work is a good way to carry on a work design project when blocked from creating system-level projects. What elements of your own work can be redesigned now, by yourself, to be healthier and to express your own values? What elements of others' work can you allow people the freedom to reconstruct outside a more formal redesign project? In fact, when an organizational preassessment indicates the organization and people are not ready for a systemwide work redesign project, these smaller efforts may be the best place to begin and may result in an organization level redesign project in the future. Gareth Morgan (1993, p. 41) sheds light on this way of creating change: "In times of change, plans and planning often prove ineffective because they create rigidities. In highly politicized contexts [dinosaur health care organizations?], they often serve as magnets for political opposition, catalyzing and crystallizing the views of those who do not want to travel in the planned direction." He suggested the metaphor of being a "strategic termite" to create change in rigid bureaucratic organizations. Being a strategic termite means creating pockets of new thinking and organization within the old, unresponsive structures. Eventually, when a critical mass is reached, newer structures will emerge. "Just do the small stuff" (Morgan, 1993, p. 49), and "Try it and see . . ." (Morgan, 1993, p. 52) are two proposed strategies that could prove successful in starting work redesign efforts in unfriendly environments. Important to doing the small stuff is finding a way to use informal communication networks to let people know what is going on and to talk about and celebrate successes.

Tracking the Process Through Research

A way to contribute to knowledge for nursing administration is to consider using a participatory action research framework (Whyte, 1991) to guide the redesign endeavor. The literature search for this chapter yielded little about the process of successful change efforts. Research reports highlighted the type of change and the degree to which it was successful, but none that were found spoke to the full process. Clearly, nurses need specific theory on the process of redesigning nursing work. Elden and Levin (1991) proposed a particularly useful model of participatory action research as a framework for work redesign. In a spirit of cogenerative learning, their model allows for creative alliances between researchers in academic settings and health care organizations. The model provides for the union of existing theory with ongoing everyday work situations. All persons are participants in designing actions that fit the institution and then in creating theory grounded in the process of creating the actions to solve everyday problems. The author found no participatory action research work redesign projects in the nursing literature. There is a desperate need for such knowledge. Currently, we are doomed to hopping on the bandwagon of work redesign, because we know change is needed and we have no research-based theory to guide us. The author also strongly recommends including the "messiness" of the process in theory development to illuminate the creative tension between what is and what could be. Such theory, based in the real world of nursing practice, would provide hope to those who wish to develop creative nursing practices within existing health care organizations.

CONCLUSION

Work is an integral part of the lives of practicing nurses. Work is not often designed to fully express the meaning of nursing, nor to create a sense of well-being for nurses and those they serve. In fact, nursing work often contributes to unhealthy levels of stress and burnout for nurses as they try to meet the ever-increasing expectations of their jobs. Although nursing work needs to be redesigned to enhance professional practice and increase productivity to contribute to organizational economic survival, the redesign efforts need to focus on preserving or re-creating the meaning of nursing work. Promoting the health and well-being of the population of nurses should be a central and guiding value for redesign efforts. Work must satisfy the soul. "How we spend our working hours—what you look at, sit on, work with—makes a difference, not only in terms of efficiency but in terms of its effect on our sense of self" (Moore, 1993, p. 7). How nursing work is designed sends a message about what it means to be a person and the value we place on the nurse as person.

Those who desire to redesign nursing work often practice in environments unfriendly to change. How can nurses, who want to make a difference by creating redesigned work in these settings, proceed? Hackman and Oldham (1980) provided some wisdom for this situation. They recognized that redesign efforts rarely find a perfectly receptive situation, and that even if diagnostics indicate a favorable climate for redesign in terms of need and readiness, efforts at system-level redesign might still need to be abandoned. As they noted, "Work redesign is probably a bad idea if those who ultimately must support and diffuse the changes *believe* it to be a bad idea" (Hackman & Oldham, 1980, p. 129). What then? Hope still exists in the following story about a young woman:

> She was walking on a long beach that was littered with thousands of starfish, which had been left there to die by the receding tide. As she walked along, she was saving their lives by picking them up one by one and depositing them back in the ocean. An older man came along and was puzzled by what she was doing. He told her that she was wasting her time because there were so many starfish on the beach that what she was doing couldn't possibly matter. She picked up a starfish to be put back in the water and turned to the man saying, "It matters to *this* starfish." (Ray, 1993, p. 291)

The message is clear. Many small efforts at redesign, such as pilot studies, trying something out to see how it works, redesigning areas of our own work in areas where we have control, thinking differently and translating that thought to action, must make a difference when such small work redesign is based in a systems perspective. Even a small change somewhere in the system will have an impact on the whole. When more of us are making small changes, the system has potential to shift. After all, if, through the efforts of many individuals, nations can be moved to change, why not nursing work in health care organizations?

REFERENCES

Ashley, J. A. (1976). *Hospitals, paternalism, and the role of the nurse.* New York: Teacher's College Press.

Beyers, M. (1991). Introduction. *Nursing Administration Quarterly, 15*(4), 43-45.

Clifford, J. C., & Horvath, K. J. (Eds.). (1990). *Advancing professional nursing practice: Innovations at Boston's Beth Israel Hospital.* New York: Springer.

Elden, M., & Levin, M. (1991). Cogenerative learning: Bringing participation into action research. In W. F. Whyte (Ed.), *Participatory action research* (pp. 127-142). Newbury Park, CA: Sage.

Hackman, J. R., & Oldham, G. R. (1980). *Work redesign*. Reading, MA: Addison-Wesley.

Kerfoot, K. (1988). "Managing" professionals: The ultimate contradiction for nurse managers. *Nursing Economics, 6*(6), 321-322.

Land, G., & Jarman, B. (1993). Moving beyond breakpoint. In M. Ray & A. Rinzler (Eds.), *The new paradigm in business: Emerging strategies for leadership and organizational change* (pp. 250-266). New York: Tarcher/Perigee.

Manthey, M. (1992). Bandwagons revisited. *Nursing Management, 23,* 20.

McCloskey, J. C. (1991). Creating an environment for success with fun, hope, and trouble. *Journal of Nursing Administration, 21*(4), 5-6.

Moore, T. M. (1993, March/April). The soul of work: Cultivating depth and sacredness in everyday life. *Business Ethics, 7,* 6-7.

Morgan, G. (1993). *Imaginization: The art of creative management.* Newbury Park, CA: Sage.

On the scene: Executive teamwork at the University of Michigan Medical Center. (1989). *Nursing Administration Quarterly, 13*(2), 43-66.

On the scene: Hoag Memorial Hospital. (1991). *Nursing Administration Quarterly, 15*(2), 39-48.

On the scene: Managed care of the Johns Hopkins Hospital. (1993). *Nursing Administration Quarterly, 17*(3), 54-79.

On the scene: Nurse empowerment for the 21st century. (1992). *Nursing Administration Quarterly, 16*(3), 20-42.

On the scene: On the move to the 21st century: Innovation and action. (1991). *Nursing Administration Quarterly, 16*(1), 22-55.

On the scene: Restructuring nursing services in the Mercy Health Services Consortium. (1991). *Nursing Administration Quarterly, 15*(4), 43-64.

On the scene: Section I—Beth Israel Hospital. (1990). *Nursing Administration Quarterly, 14*(2), 7-29.

On the scene: Section I—Riverview Medical Center. (1987). *Nursing Administration Quarterly, 11*(4), 11-35.

On the scene: Section II—University of California, San Francisco. (1987). *Nursing Administration Quarterly, 11*(4), 47-62.

Packard, N. J., Schultz, P. R., & Graham, K. J. (1993, June 5). *A population based nursing administration curriculum.* Paper presented at the meeting of the Council on Graduate Education for Administration in Nursing, Boston.

Pierce, S. F., Freund, C. M., Luikart, C., & Fondren, L. (1991). Nurses employed in nonnursing fields: Is nursing losing its best and brightest? *Journal of Nursing Administration, 21*(6), 29-34.

Porter, A. L. (1991). The consortium demonstration project planning. *Nursing Administration Quarterly, 15*(4), 45-48.

Prescott, P. A. (1986). Vacancy, stability, and turnover of registered nurses in hospitals. *Research in Nursing and Health, 9,* 51-60.

Rabkin, M. T. (1990). Ascent from mediocrity: A redefinition of nursing. In J. C. Clifford & K. J. Horvath (Eds.), *Advancing professional nursing practice: Innovations at Boston's Beth Israel Hospital* (pp. 3-13). New York: Springer.

Ray, M. (1993). Epilogue: Rebuilding the spaceship while it is still in flight. In M. Ray & A. Rinzler (Eds.), *The new paradigm in business: Emerging strategies for leadership and organizational change* (pp. 290-293). New York: Tarcher/Perigee.

Rempusheski, V. F. (1990). Constructing a conceptual model for professional nursing practice. In J. C. Clifford & K. J. Horvath (Eds.), *Advancing professional nursing practice: Innovations at Boston's Beth Israel Hospital* (pp. 282-297). New York: Springer.

Robinson, S. E., Roth, S. L., Keim, J., Levenson, M., Fleutje, J. R., & Bashor, K. (1991). Nurse burnout: Work related and demographic factors as culprits. *Research in Nursing and Health, 14*, 223-228.

Rosen, R. H. (1991). The anatomy of a healthy company. In J. Renesch (Ed.), *New traditions in business: Spirit and leadership in the 21st century* (pp. 116-128). San Francisco: Sterling & Stone.

Sanford, C., & Mang, P. (1993). A work in progress at Du Pont: The creation of a developmental organization. In M. Ray & A. Rinzler (Eds.), *The new paradigm in business: Emerging strategies for leadership and organizational change* (pp. 147-159). New York: Tarcher/Perigee.

Savage, S., Simms, L. M., Williams, R. A., & Erbin-Roesemann, M. (1993). Discovering work excitement among Navy nurses. *Nursing Economics, 11*(3), 153-161.

Senge, P. M. (1991). The leader's new work: Building learning organizations. In J. Renesch (Ed.), *New traditions in business: Spirit and leadership in the 21st century* (pp. 89-102). San Francisco: Sterling & Stone.

Simms, L. R., Erbin-Roesemann, M., Darga, A., & Coeling, H. (1990). Breaking the burnout barrier: Resurrecting work excitement in nursing. *Nursing Economics, 8*(2), 177-187.

Trofino, J. (1987). Shaping the environment for professional nursing practice. *Nursing Administration Quarterly, 11*(4), 11-12.

Trofino, J. (1992). Historical overview: Riverview Medical Center. *Nursing Administration Quarterly, 16*(3), 20-24.

van Manen, M. (1990). *Researching lived experience: Human science for an action sensitive pedagogy.* Albany, NY: SUNY Press.

Vosburgh, M. M. (1991). Product-line management through organizational redesign. *Nursing Administration Quarterly, 15*(2), 39-45.

Wheatley, M. J. (1992). *Leadership and the new science: Learning about organizations from an orderly universe.* San Francisco: Berrett-Koehler.

Whyte, W. F. (Ed.). (1991). *Participatory action research.* Newbury Park, CA: Sage.

Wise, L. C. (1993). The erosion of nursing resources: Employee withdrawal behaviors. *Research in Nursing and Health, 16*, 67-75.

CHAPTER 16

A Longitudinal Look
at Shared Governance:
Six Years of Evaluation
of Staff Perceptions

Ruth S. Ludemann
Wendy Lyons
Lisa Block

Shared governance was initiated at a 330-bed hospital in the Southwest in 1987. Following the Councilor Model, staff were encouraged to take active roles in decision making and organizational restructuring within the Nursing Division. A research team took an active role in developing an ongoing evaluation of staff perceptions of the changes. The process of change, the structural changes, and evaluation of the implementation of shared governance were documented for a 6-year period. Annual surveys of the staff were completed, with staff responding to scales that measured perceptions of organizational commitment, the work environment, degree of influence, job satisfaction, and shared governance commitment. Findings indicated that shared governance has been effective in empowering staff nurses with increased responsibility for clinical decisions and increasing positive perceptions.

AUTHORS' NOTE: The authors wish to acknowledge the contributions of Mary Hays, Vice President, Scottsdale Memorial Hospital-Osborn, and Cathleen Wilson, RN, PhD, for their assistance in implementing this project, and Joseph Hepworth, PhD, for the statistical analysis.

Shared governance, a type of work redesign, has been discussed and used in nursing for over a decade in a wide variety of forms. It became the "in" form of staff organization during the 1980s, in concert with the participative management theories of the decade. Employee empowerment and decision making at the grassroots level became a central theme for many industries, including health care. It is interesting to note that "Shared Governance" first became a topical heading in the Cumulative Index to Nursing and Allied Health Literature in 1989. Prior to that time, the few existing articles were listed under "Management." Porter-O'Grady and Finnigan (1984) were instrumental in translating participative management theories into useful practical models for nursing departments. Since that time, many hospitals have moved toward implementing a shared governance model, allowing nurses to have more autonomy as well as a greater role in decision making. Shared governance, a form of participative management, provided impetus for reorganizing and empowering nursing staffs, a change many believe was long overdue.

Although many nursing departments have now moved to a shared governance model of organization, relatively few systematic evaluations of the outcomes have been reported to date. One of the first studies (Ludemann & Brown, 1989) showed that staff perceptions were more positive after implementation of shared governance; however, a limitation of that study was that data were collected at only one point in time. Respondents were asked to recall their perceptions before and after implementation of shared governance. Another limitation was that the study was conducted 1 to 2 years after implementation, thereby not providing information regarding the changes that might have occurred over time. As both practitioners and theorists of organizational change know, major structural and cultural changes do not occur rapidly. Porter-O'Grady (1993) recently argued that real change may take at least 5 to 6 years to occur. It becomes important to study and document change over time if one is to understand the outcomes of any work redesign project.

When the nursing administration leaders and the nursing staff at Scottsdale Memorial Hospital-Osborn (SMH-O), an acute care hospital in Scottsdale, Arizona, decided to implement shared governance in the Nursing Division, they also decided to evaluate the project over time. A research committee was charged with the responsibility of developing an evaluation plan. The purpose of this chapter is twofold: first, to describe the processes that occurred during the implementation and the structure that has evolved; and second, to describe the findings that have been collected over the past 6 years to give one organization's answer to the question, "Is shared governance effective?"

Responsibility, authority, accountability, and autonomy are the driving forces of a shared governance model. The SMH-O framework was developed in response to an identified need for staff nurses to control their clinical practice. The shared governance structure was built on the basic principles of trust, individuals' needs to make contributions and have a sense of purpose, point-of-care decision making, changing job roles and responsibilities, and the equal valuing and appreciation of all levels of work.

SMH-O embarked on the journey to implementation of shared governance in August 1986. SMH-O is a 332-bed, Level I trauma, full-service hospital, offering adult health, critical care, maternal child health, and surgery services. Within the hospital is a 30-bed skilled nursing facility and a 16-bed rehabilitation unit. A conscious decision was made by senior nursing administrative staff to investigate and implement a form of participative management. Key factors leading to this decision were recruitment and retention issues and enhancement of quality practice standards.

EVOLUTION OF PROCESS

Establishing Goals

The Nursing Administrative Team began the investigation and implementation process by defining the goals of shared governance for the organization. Promoting organizational commitment was foremost. SMH-O already had a commitment to participative management. By providing an environment in which nurses could be more involved in making clinical decisions that affect nursing practice, the goal was to promote pride in being members of the Nursing Division, as well as to promote professional commitment. Encouraging full staff participation in clinical decisions was the second goal. The plan was to move clinical decision making to the unit level. Defining the concept of nursing at SMH-O was an important third goal. From this concept analysis, a nursing philosophy and nursing standards were born. Balancing autonomy and direction by defining shared decision making for clinical practice proved to be one of the most difficult goals to attain. Providing an equilibrium in managerial decision making engaged in by management and clinical decision making engaged in by practicing nurses was also a desired outcome. In clarifying the purpose, the objective was to stimulate nurses to a commitment to quality patient care in the organization. The fourth goal, encouraging individual growth, was the most exciting. Observing staff nurse leaders develop and take advantage of opportunities to professionally succeed made the efforts worthwhile. The final goal of refining the information and communication networks in a complex organization has been an ongoing challenge. All nurses must have access to the same information in order to make clinical decisions.

The first major administrative decision related to the scope of decision making and the limits of authority for that decision by staff nurses. A model for clinical practice decisions and assuring and evaluating care delivered (quality improvement) was operationalized. Functional responsibility, authority, and accountability for delivering quality patient care constituted the level of authority given to the staff. Staff nurses have the responsibility to make decisions and act on them in the area of clinical practice, and to determine the method for monitoring and evaluating their practice.

Gaining Support

Once nursing administration had defined the model with written goals and expected outcomes, hospital administration as well as board of director support was sought and granted. A consultant assisted with development of the plan and made yearly visits to evaluate progress and encourage moving to the next step.

Key questions arose as the design process unfolded. Several questions or issues were frequently asked by the implementation groups. How is support from nursing administration and hospital administration ensured in this change? The question reflects the basic trust issue. Having had a participative management structure in place prior to shared governance helped to ensure risk-taking behaviors and reinforce trusting relationships. The majority of the initial planning occurred in group settings. Group rules were established, creating a nonthreatening climate, fostering individual growth, and providing an arena for open discussion and process evaluation.

A second question frequently asked was, Who is responsible for educating other departments and the community about shared governance? Nursing administration was instrumental in communication with other clinical departments about the decision-making structure changes. The vice president of Nursing informed hospital administration of changes and process improvements. Reports regarding the change process and progress were provided to the staff. As the restructure matured, clinical support departments were included in the decision-making process and in fact, participated on the councils. The medical staff was made aware of changes on an as-needed basis, and their input was sought in decisions directly related to their ability to care for patients.

The use of change theory is an integral component of any work redesign process. Nurse managers and clinical leaders requested more skill and knowledge in instituting change. In retrospect, more structured education in change theory, given the impact of a major work redesign and change in management philosophy, warrants a high priority; rumors occur and anxiety is high during change. Communication mechanisms must be established to ensure accurate, timely information, a never-ending process. Communication in a shared governance structure becomes more complex than in the traditional hierarchical structure: Vertical, horizontal, and perpendicular information strategies need to be developed using a variety of methods to ensure communication across nursing units, nursing services, and nursing work shifts.

Selecting a Shared Governance Structure

The model selected for the implementation of shared governance at SMH-O is the Councilor Model outlined by Porter-O'Grady and Finnigan (1984). It involves a five-council structure, with four working councils overseen by the Nursing Executive Council. The Council on Nursing Education focuses on staff development, education, and improving communication patterns and mechanisms. The Council on Nursing Management manages fiscal and human resources and handles interdepartmental issues. This council supports shared governance processes at the unit level, facilitates staff accountability for decision making, and integrates decisions of other councils into the work of the Nursing Division. The Council on Nursing Practice develops clinical practice standards and defines nursing practice at SMH-O. The Council on Nursing Quality Improvement monitors standards of care and standards of practice through the nursing quality improvement program. Recommendations for changes in practice are made on the basis of monitoring and evaluation activities. The Nursing Executive Council acts as the ultimate decision-making body and coordinates the business of the Nursing Division. The council supports systemwide programs and processes.

EVOLUTION OF STRUCTURE

The evolutionary process for shared governance began in 1985 with an existing structure of eight subgroups overseen by the Nursing Quality Assurance Review Committee. The "Committee on Committees" was developed, and the skeleton shared governance framework was created with six initial work groups. Members of each work group were appointed by nursing administration.

Each group had a specific focus: (a) peer review and performance evaluation, (b) nursing practice, (c) quality assurance, (d) documentation, (e) patient education and staff development, and (f) nursing administration. Each group also had several subcommittees with assigned tasks. As the staff became more involved with participation in various groups and subcommittees, the structure was altered to encompass the new decision-making responsibilities. An example of the transition from a committee structure to a councilor structure can be seen by tracing the history of one group. Group V's original focus was on patient education and staff development. In August 1987, patient education became a part of the nursing practice group. The staff development group was retitled the Education Committee, with a primary goal of staff education. Two years later (1989), the committee became the Council on Nursing Education. At that time, two subcommittees were formed: a Legislative Task Force and Nursing Update, which was responsible for publishing a quarterly news publication for the Nursing Division. In 1990, two more subcommittees were formed: Nursing Orientation and Nursing Scholarship. At the same time, the council dissolved the Legislative Task Force and the Nursing Update Subcommittees, taking on those goals themselves. A similar pattern of committee restructuring through to council formation occurred with each group as staff claimed more responsibility for work formerly associated with management. By 1993, approximately 50% of the nursing staff actively participated in some committee decision making. Figure 16.1 depicts the present structure.

COUNCIL OUTCOMES

Although initially much of the council and committee work was directed at conceptually visualizing the structure and discussing pros and cons of communication patterns and decision-making models, each of the councils has made outstanding contributions to improved care and to enhancing the professional environment.

The Council on Nursing Practice created the SMH Nursing Philosophy and Conceptual Framework. An entirely new nursing documentation system was developed, along with a complete reorganization of the Standards of Practice and Standards of Care. Job descriptions and performance standards have been written for all levels within the Nursing Division. The Patient Education Subcommittee established a schedule of educational videos for the hospital closed-circuit television channel. Pharmacy and Laboratory managers are now members of this council.

The Council on Nursing Quality Improvement has worked to significantly reduce the percentage of patient falls and has achieved a 62% reduction in peripheral IV infections over a 3-year period. The Nursing Quality Improvement (QI) Program has served as a template for other hospital departments. The council works with unit-based QI committees and is responsible for quarterly trending of monitor results as well as trending of sentinel events and patient satisfaction surveys. A performance evaluation tool for the nursing staff was developed on the basis of the job descriptions.

The Council on Nursing Education conducts an annual needs assessment/ analysis and develops a yearly staff education plan based on the results. The

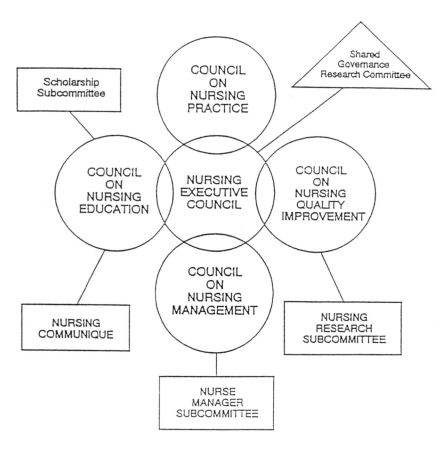

Figure 16.1. Professional Accountability Model—1993 Shared Governance Councils/Subcommittees

council has developed criteria for attendance at out-of-hospital educational programs and has also devised contracts outlining length of commitment in return for extensive in-hospital education. Nursing orientation content for new employees was totally revised, and content is presented by nursing staff. *Nursing Update,* a quarterly publication for the nursing staff, is published by the council. An additional subcommittee distributes nursing scholarship monies to qualified applicants. Many innovative speakers and workshops have been sponsored.

The Council on Nursing Management has established the Standards of Governance for the Division of Nursing. A shared governance brochure was developed by the Recruitment and Retention Subcommittee. Career fairs have been provided. Student nurse activity/clinical experiences are overseen by this council in conjunction with the Council on Nursing Education. In their interdepartment facilitation capacity, the Management Council has assisted in the implementation of decentralized support services.

The Nursing Executive Council is composed of the chairs of the councils, the vice president of Nursing, and the chairperson. Through the work of the Nursing Executive Council (NEC), the Nursing Division received accreditation without contingency during the last survey of the Joint Commission on Accreditation of Healthcare Organizations (1991). A new nursing computer network was implemented based on recommendations from a nursing task force. The council oversees and directs the work of the Shared Governance Research Committee. All members of the council serve on the Physician-Nurse Liaison Committee. Annual Excellence in Nursing Awards are presented by the council.

EVALUATION

The Research Committee first met in 1985 with the goal of designing a research project to evaluate the change to shared governance. Because the purpose of implementing shared governance was to empower the nursing staff, staff perceptions were decided upon as the critical variables. The design was a longitudinal survey with data collected annually each spring. The instrument used was the Nurse Opinion Questionnaire (NOQ), originally developed by Ludemann in 1982 and published in 1992. The NOQ is composed of five scales: organizational commitment, work environment, influence of the Nursing Division, job satisfaction, and commitment to shared governance and demographic characteristics is included (Ludemann, 1992). The NOQ was previously used in a study completed at Rose Medical Center in Denver, Colorado (Ludemann & Brown, 1989). Reliability coefficients for the scales ranged from .89 to .95. A theoretical model for predictors of perceptions of shared governance is depicted in Figure 16.2.

The five scales imbedded in the questionnaire are:

1. *Organizational Commitment,* a scale originally developed by Mowday, Steers, and Porter (1979), has been used extensively and was incorporated into the questionnaire with the author's permission. Sample item: I feel very little loyalty to this organization.

2. *Work Environment* was developed by the research team at Rose Medical Center, modifying a scale originally developed by Welsch and LaVan (1981). The instrument was reduced from a 41-item scale to an 18-item scale after a factor analysis. The scale measures attitudes toward the work environment, including percep-

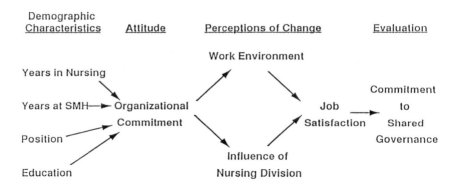

Figure 16.2. Theoretical Model for Predictors of Perceptions of Shared Governance

tions of autonomy, climate for innovation, and ability to accomplish work. Sample item: If I make a suggestion in decision making it is usually considered.

3. *Influence of the Nursing Division* was developed by the research team at Rose Medical Center, and measures perceptions of the degree of influence staff believe they have on various components within the organization. Sample item: How much influence does the staff have: With hospital administration?

4. *Job Satisfaction* was developed by the research team at Rose Medical Center and modified by the Research Committee at Scottsdale Memorial Hospital; both extrinsic and intrinsic rewards were included. Sample item: How satisfied are you with: The feeling of worthwhile accomplishment in your job?

5. *Commitment to Shared Governance* was developed by the research team at Rose Medical Center, with items paralleling items from the Organizational Commitment Scale; the only difference for most items was changing the wording to ask respondents about their attitude toward shared governance instead of asking about their attitude toward the organization. Sample item: I really care about the fate of shared governance.

Table 16.1 demonstrates the reliability coefficients for each of the years using Cronbach's alpha. Reliability coefficients have consistently been satisfactory for most of the scales, with most remaining above .8.

In addition to the scales, three open-ended questions were included, asking for respondents' perceptions of the major benefits as well as the major disappointments of shared governance and their suggestions for improvements. Responses were categorized, with interrater reliability coefficients above the .95 level. Major benefits were categorized into the following: access to information, control over practice, quality of patient care, and no perceived benefits. Categories for major disappointments included slow decision making, lack of peer/management support and commitment, insufficient time to accomplish

TABLE 16.1   Reliability Coefficients of Scales (Cronbach's Alpha)

	1986	1987	1988	1989	1990	1991	1992
Organizational commitment (15 items)	.91	.94	.90	.93	.93	.93	.91
Work environment (18 items)	.89	.74	.83	.79	.76	.88	.82
Influence (8 items)	.95	.95	.90	.84	.88	.90	.90
Job satisfaction (13 items)	.93	.90	.89	.91	.90	.90	.91
Shared governance commitment (14 items)	.90	.87	.84	.86	.91	.90	.90

work, ineffective communication, perceived negative impact on patient care, little staff decision making, and no disappointments. Categories for suggestions for improvement included improving meeting convenience and coverage, communication processes, and role clarification, shortening decision-making time, providing recognition for involvement, and educating staff about shared governance.

Each full-time and part-time RN employed by the hospital received a copy of the questionnaire annually. The response rate averaged approximately 25% per year, ($N = 100$-122), with the exception of the last year, when a 45% ($N = 188$) response rate was achieved. The majority of the respondents (approximately 90%) were employed in staff positions, with the remainder being in mid-level management positions. The average age was 38 to 40, with the average number of years employed in nursing ranging from 13 to 15, and the average number of years employed at SMH-O ranging from 6 to 10. The educational profile of respondents remained similar for each of the years, with approximately 33% of the staff having an associate degree, 33% having a BSN degree, and 20% having a hospital diploma. The remaining group had either a master's degree in nursing or a degree in another discipline. Comparable demographic profiles for the entire nursing staff were not available, so that comparisons between respondents and nonrespondents were not possible. However, nursing administrators believed that the respondent group was relatively representative of the total staff. Support for their belief was found in the last year of the data collection: No differences existed between the 25% returns and the 45% returns.

How did the professional nursing staff perceive the change to shared governance? Figure 16.3 depicts the mean scores for each year by the major variables. A clear pattern emerged. Scores in 1987, before shared governance

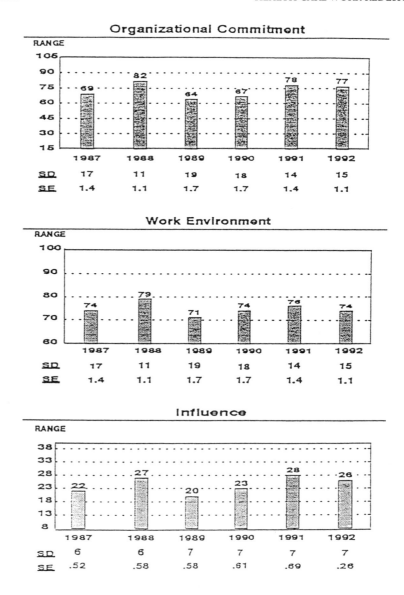

Figure 16.3. Nursing Staff's Attitudes Before and After Shared Governance

was implemented, provided a baseline profile of attitudes. All perceptions were significantly improved in Year 2 (1988), when staff were first becoming a part of the new structure. In response to the question relating to major benefits, a

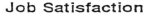

Job Satisfaction

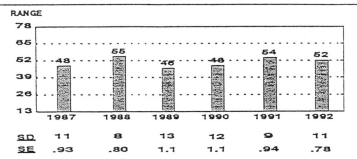

Commitment to Shared Governance

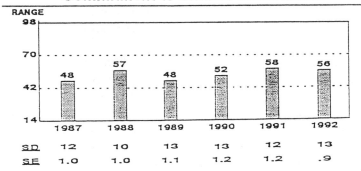

Figure 16.3. (Continued)

significant increase was noted in the nurses' perception of having more control over practice. Retrospectively, this period may be viewed as the "honeymoon" phase; staff nurses were excited with their new decision-making responsibilities via the new committee structure. They were empowered more than ever before.

A similar dramatic change occurred in Year 3 (1989), when the scores fell below the baselines of Year 1. During this year, a conflict between staff and administration occurred. Precisely at the time when staff were feeling that progress was being made toward becoming autonomous, the hospital administration announced a restructuring of the benefit package for all employees. Though the decision belonged to Administration, the methods used to communicate the changes did not follow hospital norms, leading to staff disappointment. Unionization attempts were made; attempts were subsequently voted down. The responses to open-ended questions about control over practice as a major benefit dropped dramatically. "Little staff decision making" emerged as a major disappointment. This category had not been an issue the previous 2 years. However, hospital administration did listen to the voices of the staff. New communication lines were created. Retrospectively, the third year may be viewed as the "hurt" phase; staff, with rising expectations, were let down, and some questioned the value of shared governance.

During the fourth year (1990), following resolution of the union issue and complete development of the councilor model, perceptions began to be more positive again and returned approximately to baseline level. Organizational Commitment was at 67, with a baseline of 69. Scores on both Work Environment (74) and Job Satisfaction (48) were the same as in the baseline year. Influence was increased slightly, from 22 to 23. The largest increase was in Commitment to Shared Governance, from 48 to 52. The responses to the open-ended questions validated the findings from the scales, returning to baseline values. The fourth year was therefore characterized as the "recovery" phase.

Shared governance was functioning fully in the fifth year (1991), and scores were similar to those of the "honeymoon" phase. Commitment to Shared Governance achieved the highest score of all years, 58. Fifty percent of the respondents listed control over practice as the major benefit of shared governance. Only 7% listed "little staff decision making" as a major disappointment. The fifth year may best described as the "commitment" phase. Staff were pleased with the direction shared governance was taking them, and participation was more complete. There was a sense of empowerment as well as a shared belief that the new structure was permanent.

The scores were slightly lower again in the sixth year (1992). No factors could be clearly identified to explain this finding. In response to the question regarding major disappointments, the amount of time required for decisions to be made and carried out declined annually, with a low of 10% in year 6. The research team has hypothesized that this may be the "settling in" phase, and that perceptions may not be altered more. The changes in attitudes that resulted from implementation of shared governance have peaked with the total integration of the structure. Any future changes in perceptions may be a result of changes unrelated to shared governance.

Analysis of variance was used to assess significant differences over the years for each variable. A significant F test was found for each, including commitment to shared governance, $F(5, 781) = 14.27, p < .0001$. The results of a post

TABLE 16.2   Significant Differences by Year Commitment to Shared Governance

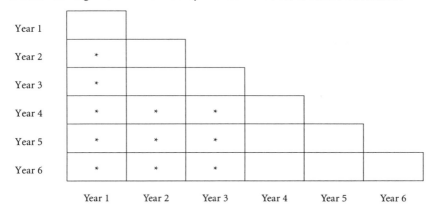

	Year 1	Year 2	Year 3	Year 4	Year 5	Year 6
Year 1						
Year 2	*					
Year 3	*					
Year 4	*	*	*			
Year 5	*	*	*			
Year 6	*	*	*			

hoc comparison for commitment to shared governance, following the ANOVA, are found in Table 16.2. Similar patterns existed for the other scales.

A few comments should be made about the theoretical model. Path analysis, using multiple regression, was performed for each year. Although space limitations do not permit description of the results of each regression, several findings of interest can be summarized:

1. Demographic characteristics, including education and age, had no predictive value in explaining the total variance of organizational commitment.

2. Job satisfaction acted as an important mediator between commitment to shared governance and organizational commitment.

3. The total explained variance for each year was as follows:

Year	Phase	R^2
1	(Baseline)	.18
2	(Honeymoon)	.11
3	(Hurt)	.45
4	(Recovery)	.24
5	(Commitment)	.42
6	(Settling In)	.38

These results have two interesting implications: First, there is greater support for the proposed theoretical model when staff attitudes are stronger, albeit in either a positive direction (Years 5 and 6) or a negative direction (Year 3); second, studies that examine attitudes or organizations at only one point in time may not confirm or negate the potential usefulness of a theoretical model. The value of a model is better determined when studied with multiple data sets.

ISSUES AND CONCERNS

Is shared governance effective in improving nurses' perceptions? The findings of this study indicate that perceptions were more positive as participation was increased. However, although the changes were in the anticipated positive direction, the degree of the changes in perceptions was less than anticipated. Several limitations of the study may serve as partial explanations: (a) the response rate for each year was limited, and (b) the sample for each year was self-selected. Not all staff chose to participate in either the study or the activities of the councils and committees, for reasons unknown. Shared governance appears to provide one solution to increasing professional accountability but may not be the total answer to increasing staff empowerment or changing attitudes. Is it possible that layering of additional motivational models, for example, implementation of quality management programs, would further improve professionalism? Further studies are needed.

Issues related to productivity and cost-effectiveness must also be examined, particularly in view of the current status of American health care reform. Costs associated with implementation of shared governance are high initially, as staff spend more time in meetings and consequently less time at the bedside. Although they are meeting to enhance their practice and subsequent service provided to patients, the cost remains. Institutions must seek and employ every method to streamline communication and decision-making processes. Structures must be developed to meet the needs of the institution, its practitioners, and its customers. In a cost-comparison study conducted by a senior nursing administrator, a 9-month savings of $194,835 was realized by restructuring the Council on Nursing Management (Pendergast, 1993).

The original Council on Nursing Management included the vice president of Nursing, the director of nurses for the Skilled Nursing Facility, the chair of NEC, all nurse managers, all clinical directors, all nursing supervisors, and a charge nurse representative. The average meeting attendance was 20. The restructuring that occurred in 1992 reduced the council size to six. The new representative council consists of the vice president of Nursing, the chair of NEC, one clinical director, one nurse manager, one nursing supervisor, and a charge nurse. A Nurse Manager Subcommittee was created and functions as the work group for the council. The membership includes all nurse managers and the director of nurses for the Skilled Nursing Facility. Meeting time has been substantially reduced from four meetings every other week to a single

TABLE 16.3   Cost Savings Realized by Restructuring of Council on Nursing
Management

	Number of Attendees	Number of Hours	Average Salary	Total
Sept. 1991–May 1992 Original Structure	243	50	$25	$303,750
Sept. 1992–May 1993 Representative Structure	45	16	$25	$ 18,000
Oct. 1992–May 1993 Nurse Manager Subcommittee	145	28.5	$22	$ 90,915
9-month savings due to restructuring:				$194,835

2-hour council meeting and a 1-hour Nurse Manager Subcommittee meeting
monthly. Meeting time alone has been reduced by 5 hours per month (see Table
16.3).

A third issue relates to defining which decisions are to be shared, or how
much will be "shared" with staff. Once the breadth of decision making has been
determined, whether solely clinical or clinical/quality, or clinical/quality/work
environment, the staff must clearly understand which decisions are shared and
which decisions are not. Without clear delineation of decision-making authority, misperceptions, mistrust, and anger result when decisions are made without staff input. At SMH-O, work environment decisions—for example, issues
related to pay and work hours—were defined as belonging to administration,
whereas decisions related to clinical practice and quality of care were to be made
by the nursing staff. Precise communication about decision-making criteria
must be an integral part of any preparatory discussions about implementation
of a shared governance structure. Accountabilties must be clearly distinguished
(Porter-O'Grady, 1993).

A fourth issue that has often been questioned is whether shared governance
can be effective if it is not a total department or organizational effort. For
example, can it be implemented on only one or two units? Our experience
indicates the necessity of having total administrative support, extending at least
from the chief executive officer, if not from the board of trustees. Some
autonomy and decision making is certainly possible at the unit level; however,
a complete Councilor Model would require that the total department be
involved. SMH-O is now planning for inclusion of other clinical departments
in a model of shared governance that would encompass the total organization.
Such a structure follows from the concepts of team management advocated by

Senge (1990) and has likewise been advocated for health care management (Kerfoot, 1991; O'Malley, 1992).

Finally, what other outcome measures need to be considered in future studies? Turnover and vacancy rates would provide data; however, their reliability may be questionable, given the cycle of the nursing shortage. Perhaps better measurements are related to professionalism and patient outcomes. The information gleaned from the open-ended questions discussed earlier has shown the true evolution of professionalism, decision making, and patient care. The time span from implementation in 1986 to the current status in 1993 indicates professionalism moving from simply sharing ideas and networking to promoting nursing as a career, to pride in the progressive and innovative nursing services provided to patients.

Initially, staff perceived decision-making authority for simple nursing care issues only. Today these nurses are taking ownership of their decisions related to determining and regulating the scope of nursing practice at SMH-O. Their involvement in the decision-making process evolved from perceiving their influence in decision making to making decisions for professional growth. On the patient care side, they moved from making responsible decisions regarding care issues to creating a work environment that reflects how nurses practice and a dedication to quality patient care. Shared governance has proven to be effective at SMH-O.

REFERENCES

Kerfoot, K. (1991). From shared governance in nursing to integrated patient care teams. *Aspen's Advisor for Nurse Executives, 7*(1), 1, 5-6.

Ludemann, R., & Brown, C. (1989). Staff perceptions of shared governance. *Nursing Administration Quarterly, 13*(4), 49-56.

Ludemann, R. (1992). Nurse opinion questionnaire. In T. Porter-O'Grady (Ed.), *Shared governance implementation manual* (pp. 118-131). St. Louis, MO: Mosby-Year Book.

Mowday, R., Steers, R., & Porter, I. (1979). The measure of organizational commitment. *Journal of Vocational Behavior, 14*, 224-247.

O'Malley, J. (1992). Organizational empowerment: Moving shared governance beyond nursing. *Aspen's Advisor for Nurse Executives, 7*(12), 1, 4-5.

Pendergast, D. (1993). *Council on nursing management, annual report, 1992-1993* (Nursing Division Annual Report). Scottsdale, AZ: Scottsdale Memorial Hospital-Osborn.

Porter-O'Grady, T. (1993). Patient-focused care service models and nursing: Perils and possibilities. *Journal of Nursing Administration, 23*(3), 7-8, 15.

Porter-O'Grady, T., & Finnigan, S. (1984). *Shared governance for nursing.* Rockville, MD: Aspen.

Senge, P. (1990). *The fifth discipline.* New York: Doubleday.

Welsch, H., & LaVan, H. (1981). Inter-relationships between organizational commitment and job characteristics, job satisfaction, professional behavior, and organizational climate. *Human Relations, 24*, 1079-1089.

CHAPTER 17

Assuming Leadership: Creating Our Future

Karleen Kerfoot

We are in the midst of one of the largest reorganizations of a business since the industrial revolution. Health care is being converted from "Mom and Pop" businesses made up of small inefficient physicians' offices, community health services, and hospitals to large corporate chains of vertically and horizontally integrated networks and processes. Buy-outs, mergers, alliances, and closures have become common in health care as the industry is restabilizing under new integrated models. Freestanding ambulatory surgery centers with attached short-stay hospital units and freestanding subacute units that specialize in, for example, long-term pulmonary or neonatal patients have been established and are examples of the innovative restructuring that is happening in health care. The proliferation of home health care providers in the 1980s continues but is taking on a new look. Models for including long-term care options are emerging in progressive communities. Market forces are driving new models of contracting for health care, and the payers are now replacing hospitals and doctors as the movers and shakers of this revolution. Reimbursement has changed from a cost-based, procedure-based methodology to new models of prepaid, capitated dollars based on subscribed lives.

New models of reimbursement are requiring that new models of practice be developed to meet this challenge. Instead of reimbursements being distributed after procedures are performed on ill patients, a system of incentives will be in place to help keep people healthy. Under capitated systems that focus on subscribed lives in integrated health systems, we will be celebrating empty hospital beds and healthy people. A whole new language of acronyms has evolved to describe arrangements such as IPAs, PHOs, and HMOs. No other segment of America has undergone such radical restructuring in such a relatively short period of time as in the health care industry. The legislation of health care reform promises to bring even more chaos to this industry.

Health care will never be the same again. There will be no going back. Moving into this era of health care will be akin to taking up residency in a different and strange country. New processes, new languages, and new paradigms are fast replacing what has become familiar to us in health care over the past few years.

Health care is long overdue for radical reengineering. Hospitals have been modeled on industrial, blue-collar, assembly-line concepts, in that patients moved through a series of units to be cared for by a discrete group of specialists and subspecialists who did not communicate with each other. Patients encountered a new set of strangers as they were transported to a new department for tests or were transferred between units. A nurse only cared for the patient during an episode of the illness and only on a discrete unit. Because of the design of the system, no system has been in place to help this nurse become aware of the outcomes of the nursing care. Facilities and processes have been built upon single-function jobs in which a large cadre of people have been trained as highly specialized professionals, such as EKG technicians. The norm in health care has become layers of hospital bureaucracy made up of people who do not talk to each other. Illness has been the organizing framework for our illness care system because money has not been available for health and prevention activities. With health care being forced to reorganize around health instead of illness, and health care facilities being forced to reorganize around new models of contracting, very little is familiar in today's health care environment.

With this new reality of health care, revolutionary changes must obviously be made. Several of the chapters in this edition have spoken to the issue of the radical redesign and reengineering of the processes and roles in health care. Reengineering, to be effective, must start with a clean sheet of paper and build models and processes on what should be, rather than revising and improving on what is (Hammer & Champy, 1993). Radical rethinking of all we do in health care is leading us to change the basic core of the structures and functions of care. Our challenge is to change the very essence of what we have been doing in order to meet the challenge of a world of health care that has been turned upside down. We will be "learning while driving" because the way that we must drive and travel for the next decade is not clear yet. To improve on what we have done in the past will not meet the challenge of this new era. We must see this new era of health care as a new model, a new paradigm.

Innovative, creative, and unencumbered thinking is the kind of innovative mentality we need for this new era of health care. The leaders of today who will serve in the future will be the ones who can develop the innovative cultures that will spawn the new models that will become the foundation of this radical corporatization of health care. Creative people who can wipe the slate clean of everything that they have ever known about health care in order to build new visions will be in great demand for this new era. Nurses must position themselves to become the keystone of these changes and to build the models that will move from nursing care to integrated patient-care models.

A NEW FRAME OF REFERENCE

"Out-of-the-box thinking" will be necessary for the nurse of the future who can think and work beyond the boxes on the organizational chart and visualize health care on a continuum. No longer will it be sufficient for nurses to think just in terms of the nursing division box in their organization. In order to develop and deliver the high-quality care that is necessary, the nurse in this new era of health care will need to switch from thinking about nursing care to thinking about planning and implementing multidisciplinary patient care that crosses organizational boundaries, divisions, and facilities. Seamless delivery systems that follow the patient through wellness, illness, and prevention will be dependent on the integration of many disciplines. Health care must appear to the consumer to be free of walls, boundaries, and speed bumps. Horizontal management models (Denton, 1991) in which nurses, managers, and leaders work across boundaries, departments, divisions, and facilities will be the norm in integrated health care systems. Gone will be the hours taken to negotiate around the walls of the bureaucracy and through layers of management. Instead, decisions will be made close to the customer by front-line people who are empowered to take on what has been traditionally thought to be the job of the manager.

Health care redesign must focus not just on reengineering the structure of the care delivery process. By envisioning the desired/ideal outcome and designing backwards, new models of efficient and effective health care systems can be designed to meet the challenges of this new era of health care. Outcome management reengineers the care delivery process around desired outcomes, not the process we have been traditionally taught (Kerfoot & Luquire, 1993; Luquire, 1993, 1994).

Tom Peters, in his book *Liberation Management* (1992), stresses that in successful organizations, frontline people are empowered and liberated to turn on their intellect and creative energy to think through new solutions. Several chapters in this volume have spoken to the issue of shared governance. The profession of nursing took a leadership position many years ago and developed empowered models of shared governance long before business and industry were thinking in these terms. Shared governance models do in fact liberate the people on the front line to think, create, and make decisions based on the customer. This creates efficiency and provides a higher level of quality. The frontline people who work in shared governance settings are no longer over-managed. Instead, people at the front line are responsible for the entire continuum of the work process. The labor/management split can be eliminated, and collegiality and synergy can replace the former adversarial relationships between management and labor when shared governance cultures are developed. In horizontal management, there are many new roles available for project leaders and members of cross-functional and cross-divisional teams. The key to the success of leaders in these new roles in synergized teams in shared governance models will be their ability to build teams and to empower groups to work together for the good of the whole as people learn to work outside the traditional boxes of hierarchical structures. Shared governance models that develop self-managed people and self-managed synergized teams will create the future of health care.

Organizational charts will not resemble the traditional pyramid of hierarchical arrangements. Instead, project teams and cross-divisional structures will transform the organizational chart, and shamrocks, star bursts, Eastman Chemical's pepperoni pizza chart, Pepsi Cola's inverted pyramid, and other formats will replace the elitist top-down organizational charts (Byrne, 1993). Instead of managing within boxes on the organizational chart, the new organizations of the future will be more concerned about managing between and across organizational units and structures. We will be involved in virtual corporations of temporary networks of independent organizations (Davidow & Malone, 1992) and partnership arrangements that span the continuum of health and illness. Multiskilled nurses who can work with many professions across many boundaries will be in demand.

As with any revolution, the health care revolution has implications for how we perform our work in the future, how we analyze and research new innovations, and how we educate future nurses. This has implications for how we build new knowledge and how we transmit knowledge to current and future health care providers. Although this chapter has focused on a new frame of reference for managing health care organizations, an underlying implication is that of collaboration with health service researchers and educators. Leaders in service, research, and education must work together if the reform in health care delivery is to be more than a "quick fix" that produces no new knowledge and does not incorporate the "out-of-the-box" thinking in the learning experiences of future leaders.

To achieve the combined creativity, efficiency, and quality necessary for survival as a health care provider, a new level of collaboration is needed, although this is rarely noted in the United States. It is the true partnership of health care providers representing the continuum of care needs. This type of partnership would be characterized by merging philosophies, resources, and expertise to create a new entity. It is not represented by the "buy-out, take-over" mentality. In the privatized, managed competition environment of our health care system, it will fall to individual leaders to create the level of collaboration described here. This must begin with outcomes management that starts with the end in mind and incorporates the philosophy, resources, and expertise of other providers and organizations. Eventually, collegial collaboration will infuse the entire operations of an organization, with seamless care representing not what the provider controls but what has been negotiated for the consumer.

SUMMARY

Leadership for this new world of health care will look different. Skill sets will be different. Leaders who can change the essence of what we do will be in demand (Beckhard & Pritchard, 1992). Nursing leadership must meet the challenge by encouraging those with a broad perspective to step into leadership positions so nursing can leap across boundaries and provide excellence in care on a continuum care basis.

These chapters chronicle the future of health care and provide a set of directions and avant-garde approaches to meet the new challenge. The authors in this publication are the movers and shakers designing a new era in health care. Our challenge is to position nursing in leadership roles, framing the future of our practice.

REFERENCES

Beckhard, R., & Pritchard, W. (1992). *Changing the essence: The art of creating and leading fundamental change in organizations.* San Francisco: Jossey-Bass.

Byrne, J. (1993, December 20). The horizontal corporation. *Business Week,* pp. 76-81.

Davidow, W., & Malone, M. (1992). *The virtual corporation.* New York: Harper Business.

Denton, D. (1991). *Horizontal management: Beyond total customer satisfaction.* New York: Lexington.

Hammer, M., & Champy, J. (1993). *Reengineering the corporation: A manifesto for business revolution.* New York: Harper Business.

Kerfoot, K., & Luquire, R. (1993). Case management/outcomes management: The role of the nurse manager. *Nursing Economics, 11*(5), 321-323.

Luquire, R. (1993). St. Luke's Episcopal Hospital practices outcomes management. *American Association for Respiratory Care Time, 17*(7), 62-64.

Luquire, R. (1994). Outcomes management and the staff nurse. *RN Magazine, 57*(5), 57-60.

Peters, T. (1992). *Liberation management: Necessary disorganization for the nanosecond nineties.* New York: Knopf.

Index

About the Editors

Kathleen C. Kelly, PhD, RN, is Assistant Professor at the University of Iowa College of Nursing, where she teaches two graduate courses in the master's curriculum—Nursing Administration II: Process, Roles, and Strategies, and Case Management in Health Delivery Systems. In addition, she directs the College of Nursing's Office of Continuing Education. During her career, she has served as a clinical nurse specialist in ambulatory nurse management at the University of Iowa Hospitals and Clinics, and for 8 years was Executive Director of the Visiting Nurse Association of Johnson County, Iowa. She is a past member of the board of directors of the National Association for Home Care, and is currently an executive committee member of the ANA Council for Professional Development and Education. She has been a member of the *Series on Nursing Administration* board of directors since the development of the second volume, and this volume is the third to be edited by her. Her research foci are health care systems and client participation in decision making as they relate to achieving continuity of care based on need rather than resources. Recent publications include *Medical Outcomes Studies: A Nursing Perspective and Adjunctive Executive Appointments for Faculty.*

Meridean L. Maas, PhD, RN, FAAN, is Professor in the College of Nursing at the University of Iowa and Adjunct Associate Executive in Nursing at Iowa Veterans Home, Marshalltown, Iowa. She teaches in the nursing service administration graduate programs for master's and doctoral students, specializing in long-term care administration. She is active in a number of professional organizations, including the American Nurses Association and the American Academy of Nursing. Prior to her academic career, she administered a nursing department and school of nursing in an acute care hospital, held staff development and supervisory positions in hospitals, and worked as a clinical specialist and administrator in long-term care. Her research focuses on the development and testing of nursing management and clinical interventions as well as classifications of standardized languages for nursing diagnoses, interventions, and nursing-sensitive patient outcomes. She has been principal investigator for research that has generated more than $3 million in external funding. She was principal investigator for one of the first federally funded grants awarded to a nonacademic institution to describe and evaluate the effects of implementing a shared governance model on patients and nursing staff, "Nurse Autonomy and Patient Welfare." Currently, she is principal investigator for a National Institute of Nursing (NINR)-funded 4-year grant to test the effects of a family involvement in care nursing intervention on persons institutionalized with Alzheimer's disease, with family members, and nursing staff. She is also coprincipal investigator (with Marion Johnson, PI) for a 4-year NINR-funded study to develop and test a Nursing-Sensitive Outcomes Classification (NOC). Her numerous publications include several books, journal articles, book chapters, and works on disk.

About the Contributors

Lisa Block, RN, BSN, is at Scottsdale Memorial Hospital-Osborn, Scottsdale, Arizona.

Carol A. Brooks, RN, DNSc, CNAA, is Associate Professor at the College of Nursing, Syracuse University, Syracuse, New York.

Carolyn L. Brown, PhD, RN, is Associate Professor at the School of Nursing, Barry University, Miami Shores, Florida.

Loraine Brown, BSN, RN is at the Indiana University School of Nursing and St. Vincent Health Services, Indianapolis, Indiana.

Sandra D. Cassard, ScD, is Research Associate at The Johns Hopkins University School of Nursing, Baltimore, Maryland.

Andrea Catania Cocovich, MA, BSN, RN, is Director of Nursing Education and Quality Management Services at Indiana Hospital, Indiana, Pennsylvania.

Sharon J. Coulter, MSN, MBA, is Chair, Division of Patient Care Operations, Cleveland Clinic Foundation, Cleveland, Ohio.

Vicki DeBaca, RN, MSN, is Coordinator of Nursing Education and Research, Mercy Health Care of San Diego, San Diego, California.

Virginia Del Togno-Armanasco, MN, RN, is Coordinator of Nursing Case Management, Tucson Medical Care, Tucson, Arizona.

Barbara A. Donaho, RN, MA, FAAN, is Program Director of the Strengthening Hospital Nursing: A Program to Improve Patient Care, and President/CEO, St. Anthony's Health Care Center, Inc., St. Petersburg, Florida.

Joyce L. Falco, MSN, RN, is Project Coordinator, Colorado Differentiated Practice Model, University of Colorado Health Sciences Center School of Nursing, Denver, Colorado.

Teri Ficicchy, BSN, RN, is Vice President for Surgical Services at Indiana Hospital, Indiana, Pennsylvania.

Mary L. Fisher, PhD, RN, CNAA is at the Indiana University School of Nursing and St. Vincent Health Services, Indianapolis, Indiana.

Becky Fitzgerald, BSN, RNC, is at the Indiana University School of Nursing and St. Vincent Health Services, Indianapolis, Indiana.

Susan R. Goldsmith, MS, RN, is Project Coordinator, Community of Patient Care Leaders, Harbor-UCLA Medical Center, Torrance, California.

Dorothy L. Gordon, DNSc, RN, FAAN, is Associate Dean for Graduate Programs and Research at The Johns Hopkins University School of Nursing, Baltimore, Maryland.

Julie Hall, MS, RN is at the Indiana University School of Nursing and St. Vincent Health Services, Indianapolis, Indiana.

Sue Harter, MBA, RN, is Director of Finance, Budget and Staffing, Tucson Medical Care, Tucson, Arizona.

Patricia Hillebrand, MEd, CNS, RN, is Vice President for Patient Services, Indiana Hospital, Indiana, Pennsylvania.

Judith Jones, MSN, RN, is Vice President of Nursing/Patient Services, Tucson Medical Care, Tucson, Arizona.

Katherine R. Jones, RN, PhD, FAAN, is Associate Professor at the University of Michigan, Ann Arbor, Michigan.

Maryalice Jordan-Marsh, RN, PhD, is Director of Nursing Research, Harbor-UCLA Medical Center, Torrance, California.

Paul E. Juras, PhD, CPA, is Instructor at the School of Business and Accounting, Wake Forest University, Winston-Salem, North Carolina.

Karleen Kerfoot, PhD, RN, CNAA, FAAN, is Executive Vice President, Patient Care, and Chief Nursing Officer at St. Luke's Episcopal Hospital, Houston, Texas.

Shaké Ketefian, EdD, RN, FAAN, is Professor and Director, Doctoral and Postdoctoral Studies, School of Nursing, University of Michigan, Ann Arbor, Michigan.

Mary K. Kohles, RN, MSW, is Deputy Director of the Strengthening Hospital Nursing: A Program to Improve Patient Care, St. Anthony's Health Care Center, Inc., St. Petersburg, Florida.

Linda J. Lewicki, MSN, RN, is Nursing Operations Manager, The Cleveland Clinic Foundation, Cleveland, Ohio.

Ruth S. Ludemann, PhD, RN, is Professor at the Arizona State University College of Nursing, Tempe, Arizona.

Wendy Lyons, RN, BSN, is at Quality Enhancement Services, Scottsdale Memorial Health Systems, Inc., Scottsdale, Arizona.

Connie Miller, RN, is a Nurse Researcher at the Cleveland Clinic Foundation, Cleveland, Ohio.

Marie E. Miller, PhD, RN, is Associate Professor and Director, AHEC System, University of Colorado Health Sciences Center School of Nursing, Denver, Colorado.

Peggy Nazarey, RN, MSN, is Director of Nursing and Project Director, Community of Patient Care Leaders, Harbor-UCLA Medical Center, Torrance, California.

Susan L. Peterson, MS, BSN, RN, is Manager of the Nursing Systems and Special Services, Columbia Hospital, Milwaukee, Wisconsin.

Richard Redman, PhD, RN, is Associate Professor and Director, Division of Nursing and Health Care Systems Administration Programs, School of Nursing, University of Michigan, Ann Arbor, Michigan.

Elisa Sanchez, BS, is Administrative Assistant, Community of Patient Care Leaders, Harbor-UCLA Medical Center, Torrance, California.

Nancy Sheets, RN, MSN, is Assistant Project Director of the Patient-Centered Redesign Program, Hartford Hospital, Hartford, Connecticut.

Cynthia Shirley, BSN, RN, is Patient Care Specialist, Telemetry, Indiana Hospital, Indiana, Pennsylvania.

Paula Siler, RN, MS, is Director of Professional Practice Affairs, Harbor-UCLA Medical Center, Torrance, California.

Cheryl B. Stetler, PhD, RN, FAAN, is Project Director of the Patient-Centered Redesign Program, Hartford Hospital, Hartford, Connecticut.

Jolene Tornebeni, RN, MSN, is Chief Operating Officer and Senior Vice President at Mercy Health Care of San Diego, San Diego, California.

Gail Tumulty, RN, PhD, CNAA, is Associate Professor and Coordinator, Nursing Administration, College of Nursing, University of North Carolina at Charlotte, Charlotte, North Carolina.

Carol S. Weisman, PhD, is Professor at The Johns Hopkins University School of Nursing, Baltimore, Maryland.

Rebeca Wong, PhD, is Assistant Professor at The Johns Hopkins School of Hygiene and Public Health, Baltimore, Maryland.

Christine A. Wynd, PhD, RN, is Director, Department of Nursing Research, The Cleveland Clinic Foundation, Cleveland, Ohio.

Mary Yarbrough, RN, MSHA, is President and Chief Executive Officer at Mercy Health Care of San Diego, San Diego, California.

Nashat Zuraikat, PhD, RN, is Associate Professor and Graduate Coordinator at the Department of Nursing and Allied Health Professions, Indiana University of Pennsylvania, Indiana, Pennsylvania.